Alternatives to Tranquillisers

Alternatives to Tranquillisers

John McKenna

Newleaf

Newleaf

an imprint of

Gill & Macmillan Ltd

Goldenbridge

Dublin 8

with associated companies throughout the world

© John McKenna 1999

0 7171 2706 0

Design and print origination by

O'K Graphic Design, Dublin

Printed by

ColourBooks Ltd, Dublin

This book is typeset in 11/14 pt Adobe Garamond

A CIP catalogue record for this book is available from the British Library.

This book is dedicated to my parents,
Kathleen and Robert McKenna,
who are both deceased.
You gave me the gift of life and allowed me
the freedom to grow up in a simple, natural way.
I wish you great peace and thank you
for doing the best you could.
Your loving son
John

Contents

Preface

It is easier to speak and write from the head than from the heart. I was trained as a scientist and then as a doctor and so spent the best part of ten years in university cramming facts into my head; hence, head-related activities come easily and feel safer. Through writing the book *Alternatives to Antibiotics* and through giving public talks and interviews for radio and television, I have felt the need from deep within me to speak more from what I have experienced than from what I have read and been taught in college; it's simply more truthful this way, even though it feels less safe. Theory can be quite boring whereas practical experience from what I've gone through in my own life and seen happen to my patients gives me amazing insight into the true nature or purpose of life.

I was born in Ireland of Celtic origin and because I spent the first eighteen years of my life in a relatively remote area, two miles from the nearest village and eight miles from the nearest town, I had a very simple upbringing steeped in nature and steeped in Irish culture. I grew up with an understanding of the unseen world as well as the seen world, where fairy trees, fairy rings, fairy forts and 'the little folk' were accepted and respected, where the spirit world was an integral part of the storytelling at night and where the music could stir very deep emotions and transport you away. At school I was instilled with a strong sense of my Celtic heritage — I learned the Irish language and Irish folklore and up until the age of ten I did Irish dancing. It was a normal upbringing, or so I thought, but after travelling extensively I became aware that the Irish are unique and have a very different view of the world to that of many other Europeans. The Irish understand many things, such as enjoying the present, being spontaneous, not needing to plan an event but rather just letting it happen, seeing signs which guide one's path in life and so on.

Let me give you an example. One Sunday at lunchtime I was sitting in a pub in a small village, Doolin in Co. Clare on the west coast of Ireland. There was supposed to be a music session that lunchtime — a music session is where local musicians come together and play traditional Irish music; these musicians hear about the session through the local grapevine and come when they wish and leave when they wish since a session has no fixed beginning and no end; it just happens! — but no musicians showed up. There were three nurses at the bar and they began to sing, encouraging everyone else to join in, which we all did. Then each person took a turn at singing or reciting poetry or telling a story. I don't think I've ever had a more entertaining Sunday afternoon in my life than I did that day and it was totally unplanned, purely spontaneous! Nowhere else in the world could this happen. This is what makes us Irish so unique.

Our upbringing is actually quite a spiritual one where a magical event like the one I've just described can happen. For me, being spiritual is just being oneself and allowing life to happen in a magical way instead of forcing it to happen according to some mental plan.

With this background you may understand why it is easier for me to appreciate things of the heart rather than of the head. Both have validity but where the head rules the heart, tension builds up within the person and causes much conflict and stress. The Western world is very much about the head, about making money, about 'progress'. My upbringing was very much about the opposite: it was about simplicity, about having time to converse and tell stories, about music and dance and about relating to a magical unseen world which was all around us. The reason why

I'm speaking about all of this is to give you some insight into where I am coming from and, I hope, to instil in you the need to preserve this unique way of being as a way of helping us to overcome the complexity of our lives and to say there is another way of living and seeing life. The more we speak and write and live our lives from the head, the greater our anxiety will be and the more we shall need tranquillisers; the more we live from the heart the more peace we shall know. I have lived from both of these spaces and so feel that the time has come now to speak out and say what I truly feel. So, this book will have factual material with scientific and medical references to substantiate what I'm saying but will also shed light on why we have become so dependent on drugs and how we can change that. It discusses how to get off tranquillisers but also how to deal with emotional difficulties in a more honest, more healing way. The book will cover a range of alternatives that I can speak about from personal experience, such as hypnosis, herbal medicines, homoeopathic medicines and nutrition, as well as some amazing nutritional supplements. There is also a chapter on self-help methods such as exercise, relaxation, meditation and visualisation. Overall I would like to feel that my true Celtic nature has found expression in this book and that it will calm your energy sufficiently to bring you some peace and contentment in your life.

John McKenna
January 1999

The Minor
1   Tranquillisers

Introduction

The minor tranquillisers include drugs that have both a sedative (calming) and a hypnotic (sleep-inducing) effect. As a consequence these drugs are referred to as sedative-hypnotic drugs. The main sedative-hypnotic drugs are the benzodiazepines, e.g. Valium, Ativan, Halcion, and the barbiturates, e.g. phenobarbitone, amylobarbitone.

The benzodiazepines rank as the most commonly prescribed drugs in most Western countries today. Since one in seven patients complain of insomnia and one in four patients have anxiety-related symptoms, several billion people worldwide are now or have at some time been on one of the benzodiazepines (or BZs, an abbreviation I have adopted in the text for convenience). It is an unfortunate truth that many people in our society need to 'pop a pill' before facing the day, or the night! Our society is so stress-ridden that we need pharmaceutical drugs to help us cope.

From the point of view of our children, we are giving a clear message that taking drugs is the way to solve our difficulties. This idea is being supported by the medical profession, a profession dedicated to acting in the best interests of humanity. I have met numerous patients who through no fault of their own have ended up addicted to one of the BZs simply because their family doctor prescribed it for sleeping difficulties, or stress, or whatever,. In essence, doctors are contributing to the number of drug addicts

1

by not being aware of the dangers of keeping a patient on a BZ drug and also by being unaware of the alternatives available.

The BZs

Table 1.1 lists some of the more commonly prescribed BZs with the chemical or generic name in the left-hand column and the brand or trade name in the right-hand column.

Table 1.1

Chemical name	Brand name
Alprazolam	Xanax
Amylobarbitone	Amytal
Bromazepam	Lexitan
Chlordiazepoxide	Librium
Diazepam	Valium
Flurazepam	Dalmane/Paxane
Lorazepam	Ativan
Nitrazepam	Mogadon
Oxazepam	Serenid
Temazepam	Normison
Triazolam	Halcion

Only one of the drugs in Table 1, Amytal, is a barbiturate, these having been all but replaced by the BZs. For years the barbiturates were the main sedative-hypnotic drugs and the name phenobarbitone was in common usage. However, they fell into disrepute because of certain inherent difficulties associated with them:

■ People became seriously dependent on them, making withdrawal quite painful.
■ People used them to commit suicides as in overdose they depressed the respiratory (breathing) and cardiovascular centres in the brainstem.
■ They were dangerous to use with alcohol, which had the power to potentiate the effect of these drugs, so making the combination quite lethal.

2

With the development of the BZs, which were safer, there was a strong drive to favour these, and today barbiturates are rarely used.

History of the BZs

In the mid-1950s Roche laboratories began a search for drugs with sedative-hypnotic effects which were safer than the barbiturates. By 1959 the first BZ was synthesised and patented as Librium (chlordiazepoxide is the chemical name). Four years later diazepam or Valium had been developed and patented and in clinical trials was found to be ten times more potent than Librium. Today there are thirty-nine BZs, of which Xanax (alprazolam) is the newest. They all have a strong sedative and hypnotic effect.

The BZs are often divided into short-acting and long-acting BZs. The short-acting ones have a duration of action varying from two to six hours; those are mainly used as sleeping pills. Examples are flurazepam (Dalmane or Paxane) and temazepam (Normison).

The longer-acting ones have a duration of action in the body varying from twenty-four to thirty-six hours; these are used to treat anxiety. Examples are diazepam (Valium) and oxazepam (Serenid).

Some of the BZs do not fit easily into either of these categories and so are often called medium-acting. Examples are bromazepam (Lexitan) and lorazepam (Ativan). These can be used both as a sedative and as a hypnotic. This information is summarised in Table 1.2.

Table 1.2

	Duration of action	Examples
Short-acting BZs	Two to six hours	Dalmane Normison
Long-acting BZs	Twenty-four to thirty-six hours	Valium Serenid
Medium-acting BZs	Eight to twenty hours	Lexitan Ativan

Uses of the BZs

The BZs have a wide range of uses in clinical medicine, as can be seen in Table 1.3. Their main usage is as sedatives. Sedative drugs moderate excitement, decrease activity and induce calmness. Hence, if you are under stress, acutely or chronically anxious, unable to cope with the difficulties of modern life or have undergone trauma, e.g. a road traffic accident, then one of the BZs will often be prescribed by your family practitioner.

Their second main usage is as hypnotic drugs. Hypnotic drugs produce drowsiness and facilitate the onset and maintenance of sleep. Hence they are the main form of sleeping tablets.

They also relax skeletal muscle and so are used to treat muscle tension in different parts of the body, especially in the lower back. Their fourth main usage is as pre-anaesthetic medication to ease the acute anxiety associated with an operation or medical investigation. They can also be used in the treatment of epilepsy.

Table 1.3

Uses of the benzodiazepines
1. Sedative — to treat anxiety
2. Hypnotic — to treat insomnia
3. Muscle relaxant — to treat muscle spasm
4. Anti-epileptic — to treat epilepsy
5. Pre-anaesthetic — to treat acute anxiety before surgery

The overuse of benzodiazepines has had far-reaching consequences for us all. It has discredited the image of the drug companies in that they are seen to be about drug-pushing, i.e. they put pressure on doctors to prescribe drugs thereby guaranteeing their profits even at the expense of people's health; it has discredited the medical profession to the point where many people are now moving away from their family doctor to doctors like myself in their search for a safer, more natural form of medicine. But I believe that perhaps the real damage has occurred in a more subtle, unseen way in that it has given a non-verbal message to our children and grandchildren that (a) it's okay to take harmful addictive drugs, and (b) it's acceptable to deal with emotional difficulties by taking drugs which numb one's emotions, making true emotional healing virtually impossible; in other words, let's suppress the emotion — e.g. anger, resentment, grief — with a drug and everything will be fine!

I believe the greatest gift that we can give our children is to show them how to heal. Our children, like us, will experience difficulties in their lives. If they have learned from you how to deal with these, by observing how you confront difficulties and heal the pain associated with them, then they will cope well in life and not need addictive drugs. However, if they see you hiding away from the pain and using drugs to support your weakness, then they will do likewise. It's no small wonder then that illicit drugs are a major problem in most modern cities today. If you want to solve the drug problem start with yourself and show your family what true healing is about.

How the BZs Work
For the BZs to calm you or help you get to sleep, they act on a particular part of the brain called the reticular formation, which controls your alert, awake, conscious state. In the reticular formation there are nerve cells and between each nerve cell are chemicals called neurotransmitters, which have an excitatory action or inhibitory effect, i.e. they either excite the next nerve cell so increasing your alert state or they inhibit or block nerve impulses so decreasing your alert state. Exercise will release excitatory neurotransmitters so making you more alert or awake; soft music will have a calming effect by increasing the level of inhibitory neurotransmitters — see Figures 1.1a and 1.1b.

Figure 1.1a

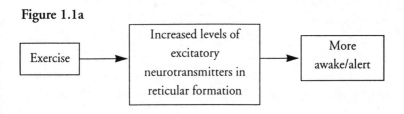

5

Figure 1.1b

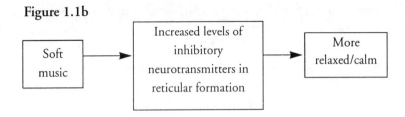

One of the most important *inhibitory* neurotransmitters in the brain is GABA (gamma-amino butyric acid); it depresses brain activity and will induce a calm and ultimately a sleep state. The mode of action of the BZs is to increase the level of GABA in the brain so inducing a calm, relaxed state. This is oversimplifying the issue because in truth there is much we still don't know about how the brain works. Many of the modern central nervous system drugs such as the BZs, Prozac and so on are used by doctors but the truth is that they have side effects which cannot be adequately explained by modern science. As regards many of the drugs given to patients, we do not understand how they work and so in truth we are prescribing blindly to some extent. The way in which some herbal medicines work is teaching us a lot about what we *don't* know (see p. 61 on kava kava and p. 65 on hypericum). These natural substances are virtually free of side effects and yet produce such powerful calming effects — clearly the above neurotransmitter model of how the BZs work is inadequate!

Side Effects of the BZs

1. EFFECTS ON THE CENTRAL NERVOUS SYSTEM

Because the BZs have a general depressive effect on brain function, they produce excessive drowsiness and as a result can impair muscle function, causing ataxia (an abnormal gait); they also impair mental function, causing intellectual dysfunction, which makes ordinary day-to-day planning difficult. They can, especially if dosage is high, cause respiratory depression and cause low blood pressure, leading to dizziness and fainting. There may be excessive salivation and depressed sexual function, i.e. reduced libido. Many patients complain of amnesia, i.e. loss of memory, affecting everything that happened from the time they swallowed the pill through to the time it was eventually excreted from the body.

2. Physical Dependence
The major side effect, however, has to do with dependence. Many patients on these drugs become physically dependent on them and are unable to stop them as the withdrawal effects are too severe. The body's chemistry alters to accommodate the BZs; once they are withdrawn the chemistry can get disturbed to the point where the calming effect of the BZs is removed but a rebound anxiety manifests, making life unbearable. At this point the patient will often start taking the pills again simply to ease the rebound anxiety. This is what physical dependence means — your body becomes physically or chemically dependent on the drug.

3. Emotional Blunting
Another major side effect associated with use of the BZs is blunting of the emotions. Many patients complain that they do not experience the normal highs or lows of life, often saying that they feel like emotional zombies. Worse still, strong emotional states such as grief at the loss of a loved one will stay suppressed until you come off these drugs.

Case History

After the death of her husband, Linda was put on Lexitan (bromazepam) and was left on this drug for a period of eight years by her local GP because each time she tried to come off it she got significant rebound anxiety. Eventually, through the help of a Chemical Dependence Unit in her local hospital she was able to get off Lexitan. It was only then that she began to experience the grief associated with the death of her husband. This is an example of how the BZs can suppress deep-felt emotions.

4. Altered Sleep Pattern

Yet another major side effect has to do with suppression of REM sleep (rapid eye movement or very deep sleep). After falling asleep, the depth of your sleep state increases until you reach a very deep state when dreaming occurs. It is often in this dream state that the body moves, facial expression changes and you get rapid eye movements (REM). After this, the sleep state becomes gradually more shallow, as shown in Figure 1.2. Then the whole cycle repeats itself, occurring in all about six times a night if your sleep is undisturbed.

Figure 1.2

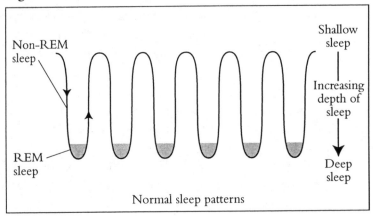

Normal sleep patterns

The BZs suppress REM sleep and if you have been on these drugs for months or years and come off them, you can suddenly get hallucinations and very vivid dreams and nightmares, even during the waking state, as the brain attempts to compensate for all the lost dreamtime. This can clearly be very disorientating for the patient.

As you can see, the side effects of these drugs are significant. Not everyone will experience side effects and some will experience only one or two of these effects while others will experience many. As a rule, however, they are not safe to use if driving, doing a very responsible job or operating dangerous equipment. The side effects will be made worse by the concomitant use of other drugs that depress brain function, such as the barbiturates, anti-depressants and alcohol.

How the BZs Interact with Other Drugs
Because a patient is often on a tranquilliser for long periods of time, the chances increase that at some point during treatment, he/she will receive another drug. It is now established that the BZs interact with a number of other drugs. If taking a BZ, do not use another sedative or anxiety-reducing drug, including alcohol, as the sedative effect can cause respiratory depression, coma and ultimately death.

The anti-ulcer drug cimetidine (Tagamet) reduces or slows down the metabolism of the BZs, so prolonging their effects in the body; this is particularly the case with chlordiazepoxide (Librium) and diazepam (Valium). Drugs which have a similar interaction with the BZs are oestrogens in the pill and hormone replacement therapy, as well as isoniazid, which is an anti-tuberculosis drug. Other drugs reduce the effects of BZs, so making them less effective. These include antacids, tobacco and another anti-TB drug called rifampin. This information is summarised in Table 1.4.

Table 1.4

Drugs which increase the effects of BZs
— Cimetidine
— Oestrogen (pill, HRT)
— Isoniazid
— Other sedatives
— Alcohol
Drugs which decrease the effects of BZs
— Antacids
— Tobacco
— Rifampin

The Elderly and the BZs

The use of the BZs in the elderly deserves special mention. The BZs are broken down by the liver and got rid of from the body via the kidneys. Both liver and kidney functions are often impaired or less efficient in the elderly. If the liver is impaired the drug will not be broken down as rapidly and so the depressive action on the brain will be prolonged. In addition, if kidney function is impaired the drug will remain in the blood for longer, possibly enhancing the side effects. If you consider the case of an elderly male patient who may have prostate enlargement which will block urinary flow as well as kidney and liver impairment, it is not hard to understand how this patient will suffer more side effects and perhaps too potent a therapeutic effect.

It is commonplace in geriatric wards in hospital for an elderly patient on admission to be given a BZ to help them relax and sleep as some elderly patients can get very anxious or disorientated when taken from familiar home surroundings into an unfamiliar hospital environment. If these patients stay in hospital for a lengthy period they then run the risk of getting hooked on these drugs and may be unable to get off them later.

Summary

The BZs are useful drugs and do have an important therapeutic role in certain limited situations such as acute trauma — surgery, road traffic accident, death of a loved one and so on. These drugs, however, have no place in the treatment of chronic anxiety or chronic insomnia. There are effective alternatives for these conditions which are safe and free of side effects. The BZs must never be used for longer than two weeks because of the serious risk of becoming physically dependent on them. They must be used with extreme caution in the case of the elderly.

Introduction

Because I have gained a reputation as a doctor who can help people deal with anxiety and depression using natural methods, I see many patients, some of them quite young, suffering from anorexia, bulimia and substance abuse. In Capetown, where I am currently living, one of the major treatment centres for eating disorders is full of young girls from high schools who suffer intense emotional pressure, both at school and at home, to perform well academically. Years ago I saw the same pattern among teenagers in Ireland preparing for the Leaving Certificate examination; many of them were young men suffering from gastritis, peptic ulcers and other gastro-intestinal problems. At that time Ireland had the highest suicide rate in Europe, especially among young people, who were under intense pressure. This pattern of self-abuse among teenagers is common in many Western countries. It is hard to respect a society that allows its youth to carry such burdens, to the point where a significant number of them either kill themselves or abuse themselves physically with drugs or by other means. Often it is the more sensitive ones who feel the pressure more acutely and who end up in difficulty. What has struck me most is that many of the younger patients I have treated over the years in Ireland and in other countries have a highly sensitive nature and a high level of self-awareness. They are so acutely sensitive that they absorb the pain and negativity of others, making it hard for them to cope with their own pain and difficulties. If this negativity is not released it turns inwards and can set up a cycle of self-abuse.

Case History — Mary: Age Thirty Years

Mary came to me to seek help with getting off tranquillisers, which she had been on since her late teens. She had grown up with a very abusive mother who had a major problem with alcohol and both prescription and street drugs. Her mother was abusive both physically and verbally, making Mary's life very painful and frightening. At the age of eighteen her family doctor prescribed a tranquilliser to help her cope with her final school exams; twelve years later she was still on the same drug. Mary was going to see a psychologist five days a week and had been doing that for six months prior to coming to see me. Before this, she had been to see a psychiatrist for anorexia and before that had been in two substance abuse clinics trying to deal with her dependence on alcohol and drugs.

What was striking about Mary was her very gentle sensitive nature. She was crying out for help at a very deep level but was clearly not getting enough as she was still in emotional and spiritual difficulty. She also had very clear insights into her difficulties but felt powerless to change her pattern of self-abuse. Through the use of acupuncture and later self-hypnosis, Mary was able to get off and stay off the tranquillisers but more importantly was able to learn to like herself and to discover the more positive aspects of her nature. With each acupuncture session I used to ask her to express her feelings as she found it hard to get in touch with her emotions. It started with her expressing how she felt when each acupuncture needle was twirled and ended up some months later with her being able to open up to the pain she felt when her mother got angry with her when drunk. Later through counselling and hypnosis she was able to forgive her mother and to explore who she was, to discover her own true nature and learn that she was quite different from her mother and so did not have to continue to absorb her mother's negativity.

Mary is now helping other people with eating disorders and chemical dependence, counselling them and practising a variety of therapies including relaxation, visualisation and aromatherapy. Her true nature is now emerging from the pain of her past and is a testimony to the fact that the beauty of being human is our ability to change at a very deep level.

Another pattern that I see among patients in my clinic is one where there is almost a split in the energy between the physical and mental bodies on one side and the emotional and spiritual bodies on the other side. Let me explain what I mean by this. I see many patients who have a high level of activity in the physical and mental bodies, i.e. they are very physically active with a whole agenda of things to get done each day and their thought processes never stop, even when they are trying to rest or sleep.

These people often make little time in their lives for expression of their feelings through talking, writing, painting, music, dance and so on, and often have difficulty exploring a loving relationship and so gaining an understanding of their spiritual needs. Communication of one's feelings and giving and receiving unconditional love are as essential for one's development as doing and thinking. Being blocked emotionally and spiritually is the root cause of much illness in the West. The next case history illustrates this point well.

Case History — Patrick: Age Fifty-Two Years

Patrick had a chronic cough for six weeks which was productive of copious amounts of yellow phlegm every morning. He also complained of excessive sweating, heart palpitations and a loose bowel motion. He was self-employed and was under a lot of financial stress.

All the medical investigations we did were normal, except that he had an overgrowth of commensal organisms in the sputum and a 3 plus overgrowth of Candida in the bowel; in other words, the good healthy protective flora of both the respiratory and the digestive systems was disturbed. We corrected this using diet and nutritional supplements and before long Patrick was physically a lot better. However, what struck me about him was his skilful ability to deflect questions relating to his childhood and to rationalise his feelings about emotional issues. He had difficulties feeling anything and was functioning purely at a physical and mental level. On exploring the details of his upbringing in Ireland it became clear why he was so blocked. Being quite sensitive he had suffered a lot emotionally at a school well known for its brutality and he was picked on quite often. I could relate well to his experiences as I was educated by equally angry and frustrated teachers. His home life was also quite difficult as he was the youngest of ten children and got little affection from either parent.

Although it was relatively easy to cure Patrick of his physical symptoms, I felt sure that they would recur at some future point. Illness has a way of not letting go of you until you heal the real source of your disease, releasing the anger and the fears which control you. Patrick was not ready to deal with this. Sure enough, six months later he was back again with the same symptoms. I treated him again and am awaiting the next recurrence. Even though I can see the cause of his illness, it is necessary to wait for him to see it also. Nature has a way of not letting you off the hook until you confront the real illness, which is often an illness of the soul.

Abusive Patterns in Western Society
The abusive patterns in our society are very obvious if one looks at television or reads a newspaper; they are filled with violence in the form of killing, raping and so on. Our society is all about abuse because it is based on and so reflects the negative side of our being — fear! It is through fear that your life as a child is controlled by parents, teachers, priests and so on, and later as an

adult you exercise the same control over others by doing unto others what has been done to you. It is rare to find people who have been able to overcome this fear and live as free spirits, not trying to play roles or conform to someone else's idea of what is acceptable and unacceptable, but just free to be themselves. Yet the truth is that we all yearn to be free. Most people cleverly entrap themselves through relationships, through work, through having children, through financial debts, so making the route to freedom very difficult and risky, but therein lies the dilemma and therein lies the challenge. I believe that the only route to happiness is by being totally free to have the time and the space to discover who you truly are and by allowing your true nature full expression. Illness can help us to achieve this by forcing us to take the time to re-examine our lives. This re-examination of our lives may be delayed or prevented by the use of drugs such as tranquillisers, which you have already learned can suppress one's emotions.

Western vs. Primitive Concepts

Having lived with very primitive people in West Africa and having been brought up in Western Europe, I have experienced two ways of viewing the world. Western society instils us with a set of concepts which are inherently false, which are opposed to the laws of Nature and which cause tremendous internal conflict in people, leading to a dependence on pharmaceutical drugs. Let me explain what I mean by that.

Below is a table (Table 2.1) with two columns which I have loosely named 'Western concepts' and 'Primitive concepts'. They outline the concepts or thinking that govern one's upbringing in these two human communities. The first concept deals with how one interacts with and views other members of the community. In the West one is taught that it is 'every man for himself', hence the tendency to compete with others whether it be at school, at work, in sport or among siblings; this leads to a greater separation between individuals and enhances any feelings of isolation or loneliness. Many years ago I lived in Canada for a short time and remember seeing three-month-old babies being left in day care centres at 7.00 a.m. and being collected at 6.00 p.m. five days a week. There is an economic pressure on mothers now to join the 'rat race' and leave their babies in foster care. The separation that a competitive thought pattern produces is now creating divisions between loved ones within a family.

In contrast, primitive people such as the Fulani in West Africa see themselves as part of a community, living in groups of fifty to a hundred people, similar to the way in which the plains Indians of North America lived. They are bound together by the elders of the tribe, who make the major decisions regarding the welfare of the community, e.g. where to make camp and when to move with the changes of season, in addition to solving interpersonal disputes and arranging special ceremonies such as burials and marriages. The elders are held in high regard by the younger members of the tribe as their wisdom and experience of life is called upon to guide the tribe; the older one gets, the greater the respect and the more elevated the position one occupies in the tribe.

Table 2.1

Western concepts	Primitive concepts
1. Every man for himself	1. Everyone is part of the community
2. Take, make and throw away	2. Take only what's needed
3. Artificial time — clocks!	3. Natural time — sun, moon, seasons
4. Everything is outside us	4. Our inner world is reflected in the external world
5. Based on money and power	5. Based on simplicity
↓	↓
Anxious people	Tranquil people

This is in sharp contrast to Western society, where the very young and the very old who are not able to *compete* are shunned by the society and put into institutions such as day care centres for the young and old age homes for the elderly. One's physical needs such as food, sanitation, etc. are met in these centres but the sense of belonging, of contributing, of being accepted, of being cared for and of being loved is often absent. There is no substitute for human love and compassion. Centres for the young and elderly have to make money to survive and this is often the primary motivation behind them.

The second point mentioned in Table 2.1 concerns one's interaction with the environment and with the planet. Our society is based on the 'take, make and throw away' concept where the driving force is profit and in some cases greed. We take things from the environment (e.g. oil), use it to make something (petrol, diesel) and then dump the waste (car fumes into the atmosphere). This is disrespectful of Nature in three ways. Firstly, we dig holes in the surface of the planet unaware that the same surface is there to feed and nourish us at many different levels. Secondly, we consume energy in the form of electricity, water and so on, which has a damaging effect on the planet, e.g. hydroelectric projects may provide electricity but cause incredible damage to Nature. Thirdly, we dump highly toxic waste materials into the atmosphere or into rivers, lakes and the sea, wreaking havoc environmentally yet again. In contrast, the Fulani live in harmony with Nature, taking only what is necessary and always giving thanks to God for what they have been provided with. The simplicity of their lifestyle and their humbleness and innocence reminded me of my own childhood in Northern Ireland. These primitive people show a great respect for Nature — seeing Nature and the planet as essential for their survival in the same way that we in the West may see money as essential for our survival.

The third point in the table refers to the concept of time. Primitive people such as the Fulani do not wear watches, do not have alarm clocks and know nothing of minutes, hours, days, months or years. Their daily clock is the sun, their monthly clock is the moon and their yearly clock is the seasons. They rise with the sun and end their day's activities as the sun sets. They do little in a day apart from washing, eating, herding cattle and taking milk in calabashes to the local market; there is a lot of time for human interaction. They are aware that time is accelerating but see no need to speed up with it. In contrast, we in the West are stressed out by our concept of time. Our lives are organised around the clock. We Irish people tend to be quite relaxed about time but other Europeans, especially the Germans, can be quite anxious about it.

When I was a teenager I used to go out with a German girl who lived close by. Her parents invited me to join them for an evening meal to celebrate their wedding anniversary. They asked me to come at 7.30 p.m. I arrived at 7.35 thinking I was on time only to find them already eating and very upset that I was five minutes late. I was shocked at their response. In my culture, we do not have the same regard for punctuality — the Irish are quite easygoing as a race of people. The Germans, as I learned that day, obey the clock almost to the point of obsession. Needless to say I did not get another invitation to supper. My girlfriend and I did not get married either!

An Irishman being interviewed on American television was asked about the Irish laid-back approach to life. The interviewer said, 'The Spanish have a word called "mañana" which means leaving things off until tomorrow. Do you have a similar term in the Irish language?' The Irishman scratched his head, thought for a few minutes, smiled and answered: 'Yes, we have about ten terms which mean the same thing but none with the same degree of urgency as "mañana".' Despite their obsession with punctuality, the Germans and many other Europeans love Ireland as it is a very relaxed, simple, human place to live.

The fourth point in the table refers to our connectedness to ourselves, to our feelings and to our own intuition. In the West we focus our attention on the outside or external world. At medical school, one is taught about infections as being caused by viruses or bacteria or fungi, for example. We have a belief that nervous disorders such as anxiety are due to external circumstances such as stress at work, the break-up of a relationship and so on. Every other culture on this planet sees disease from a very different perspective. The Fulani with whom I lived believe that one's inner world is reflected in the external environment, i.e. it is never the external event, such as work stress, that causes the disease but rather our inner response to this external event. Like the Irish, the Fulani see no separation between the seen and unseen worlds, and in some of their ceremonies — as in many Celtic ceremonies and legends — these two worlds can come close to one another as at the time of death. There is a traditional belief in Ireland that you may, if you are sensitive enough, hear the Bean Sí (woman fairy) knock on the door of a home where a family member will die. This is an example of how a member of the unseen world, a fairy in this instance, can help by forewarning you of a death. Needless to say I grew up in fear of the Bean Sí, hoping that she would never knock on our door.

Disease is not some unwelcome visitor from our environment like a bacterium or virus. Rather disease is the external or physical manifestation of an inner weakness or conflict. People who are more prone to getting viral infections such as the common cold or flu are those who are under pressure or stress; this fact has been proven scientifically in numerous studies. Disorders such as hypertension (high blood pressure) and angina are commonplace in the West but non-existent among primitive people. Asthma, eczema, hay fever, sinusitis, infections, digestive problems, bronchitis, headache and so on are alarmingly common in the West but absent for the most part among the Fulani; their main difficulty lies in parasitic infections and infections such as malaria, bilharzia, sleeping sickness, etc. They treat these disorders herbally for the most part in conjunction with spiritual healing which is performed at special healing ceremonies. They believe that diseases represent a disharmony not only in the person but more importantly between the seen and unseen worlds, i.e. between oneself and one's ancestors. Hence, treatment is not just of a

19

physical nature but also aims at reconnecting one with the non-physical world by performing a certain ritual or ceremony, e.g. slaughtering an animal.

These are clearly two very different approaches not just to the treatment of medical disorders but to dealing with the problems that beset us in life. One culture focuses on the external world, the other focuses on both the external and internal or seen and unseen worlds.

For the Fulani, like the Celts, the source of all physical life and hence all physical difficulties is in the spiritual or unseen world and so help and healing must be primarily of a spiritual nature. In Ireland we have special healers who through the laying on of hands can heal many physical ailments. Primitive people see a deeper meaning to physical difficulties; Westerners often interpret them as purely physical.

The final point mentioned in Table 2.1 relates to control, how it pervades our Western approach to everything in our lives and how remarkably absent it is among primitive peoples. In the West we are cut off from our emotions and from our real or true selves (or soul or spirit). We are taught not to trust what *we* feel but to trust and believe in what our parents, our teachers, our religious teach us. Immediately, this sets up a conflict within us. Your gut feeling may tell you one thing and your parent or teacher may tell you the opposite. Out of love and respect and in some cases fear of the parent or teacher, you suppress what your intuition is telling you and put faith in what others are saying. This is the basis for internal conflict. We then proceed to spend the rest of our lives struggling with this same basic conflict. Ultimately, your intuition or heart must speak and when it does your life undergoes dramatic change to the point of being turned upside down.

In contrast, primitive society depends for its very existence on this instinct or intuition or gut feeling and so it is encouraged in children. By the time these children are adults they are so in tune with themselves that they can feel or sense what is happening in others. They would often ask me what was in my heart but I could sense that they knew the answer and stating it was unnecessary. Primitive society needs to stay tuned to Nature to be able to survive; the people have to know if the weather is going to change, where they will find water, and so on. We in the West are so far removed from Nature that we do not need to develop this same inner sense.

For Western society to succeed, it has to control you. Would anyone willingly co-operate in their own self-destruction if they were aware of it? You must be kept distracted and kept conditioned so that you will not question the basis of Western society. You must be kept busy and distracted so that you will not have the time to question, and kept conditioned so that your belief in the cultural package is guaranteed. Today, many young people are questioning the role of many of the structures in our society — the educational system, the medical system, the church, the financial system and so on and are seeking to change these structures or just not support them. In Ireland, the stronghold that the Catholic church had on the country has been loosened, due mainly to the fact that a significant percentage of those under twenty-five no longer accept the message the church preaches. They see through the words to the base that the church is working from, which unfortunately is a base of control. The church uses fear as the means of control — fear of God, fear of Jesus, fear of the devil and so on. Any person or institution that preaches peace but practises violence is in difficulty.

Yet, one is forced to respect and support such a church by going to mass on Sundays, giving money and so on. The Catholic church is one of the wealthiest organisations on the planet and wields considerable power. Why has an organisation committed to spiritual values needed money and power? Many young people that I speak to are sick of the hypocrisy of the church and so refuse to support it; many are seeking true spiritual help not through religion but through other means.

What is interesting is that primitive communities are devoid of banks, insurance companies, police, legal system, churches, schools and so on. These people don't need any of these structures but rather live a simple, natural life and problems that arise are solved in a very humane way by the elders in the tribe. These people are in touch with themselves, with their own true nature. Their warmth and innocence and playfulness is almost childlike. Chronic anxiety, sleeplessness and depression are rare in such communities. They do not seek tranquillity (or tranquillisers!); *they are tranquil*. Westerners are not in touch with their own inner nature, nor with the natural world around them. They are divided, cut off, separated from their warm, childlike innocence and so always in conflict. This conflict is externalised in the workplace, in a marriage relationship, in other aspects of one's life. When a number of aspects of one's life get into difficulty, e.g. problems at work, divorce, loss of a loved one, the anxiety level increases, leading to the need to reach for a pill to suppress or reduce it.

Case History — John: Age Nineteen Years

I met John in 1989 in hospital in Dublin where he was being investigated for severe upper abdominal pain. On gastroscopy he was found to have severe gastritis with small ulcerations. He was treated at the time with antacids and an anti-ulcer drug, cimetidine. Three months later he was back in hospital with the same complaint. On this occasion the consultant surgeon decided to treat him with the same medication but to add a tranquilliser, Lexitan, and to refer him to a psychiatrist for assessment. The psychiatrist concluded that John was depressed and had poor coping skills at handling stress — he was preparing to sit his final school exams and was under extreme pressure from his parents to do well and get entrance to university to study medicine. The psychiatrist added an antidepressant, Zoloft, to John's medication list and referred him back to his family doctor. Two months later John was dead, having committed suicide by throwing himself in front of a moving train. John was back in hospital again but this time in the post-mortem room.

There was a crying need in John's case to deal with his stress levels in a non-drug way and to help him cope with what was obviously severe internal conflict — John's wishes versus those of his parents. This young man needed help. Do not let this happen to your child.

As you can see from Table 2.1, there is more than one way of existing on this planet. Personally, I believe that Western society must change, not just the medical system, educational system and so on, but philosophically. This can happen if we each increase our level of self-awareness and are truthful about how we feel even when the feeling conflicts with our upbringing and our cultural norms.

It is my aim while living in South Africa to open a centre devoted to raising one's level of self-awareness. The energy behind this centre must be one of love and compassion for people, not profit or boosting one's ego. The centre will be residential, with people free to come for a day, a week, a month or as long as they feel the need. It will provide a space for people to open up emotionally, where they can feel safe and comfortable and supported in releasing buried feelings such as anger or grief, where they can explore a better way of living through meditation, relaxation, visualisation, good nutrition and so on, and where conventional and alternative medical therapists become one in the name of helping people heal. I believe that if people are given a safe, supportive space and sufficient time, they will heal spontaneously. However, there is no harm in helping a person explore themselves through dance, art, music, meditation, etc. but allowing each individual the power to choose what he/she feels is right for them at that particular point in their lives. Each of us knows deep down inside what we need to do to heal — we have all the answers inside us. Hence, therapists working in such a centre need only guide; the power of decision must always reside with the person wishing to heal. Remember that there is no right or wrong way to heal — only your way!

If you would like to support the setting up of such a centre in Ireland, South Africa or anywhere in the world please write to me and let me know. My address is given at the end of this book.

Case History — Elsie: Age Thirty Years

Elsie came to see me in Capetown in October 1997. To quote her exactly, she said: 'I feel like cracking up inside as I'm under such pressure at work and at home.' From talking with her it became obvious that she was taking on everyone else's problems — her boss's problems associated with a merger, the anxieties that her workmates were experiencing about their future in the company, and her husband's financial difficulties which caused her immense strain as he was unable to sleep at night and often woke her up.

Elsie has learned what many people in the healing arts have to learn — that is, that her first responsibility is to herself and that only from a position of strength can she help others. Through becoming more aware of herself she had become aware of her limitations and communicated these to her boss, her workmates and her husband. I also used kava kava, a powerful relaxant herbal medicine, to assist her during this learning period. Today her life is much better and her inner conflict has been replaced by a greater sense of calmness and control over her life. She has learned that she is important and so must protect herself.

Summary
Stress is defined as any reaction that upsets homeostasis, which is the system in the body that keeps a constant internal environment. Stress can cause anxiety by disturbing the internal environment and in the short term can lead to insomnia, fatigue, shortness of breath, palpitations, sweating, mood changes such as irritability, hot flushes, chills, cold hands, hypoglycaemic symptoms and, as in John's case history above, gastro-intestinal symptoms such as gastritis and duodenal ulcers. In the long term,

if the stress continues, a whole range of disorders can result, including allergies, autoimmune disorders, an increased susceptibility to infections, hormonal imbalances and ultimately heart disease and cancer. Why are there such high levels of stress in Western society compared to other societies? I believe that this has to do with the fact that in the West we have moved away from Nature to a very unnatural way of life, we have moved away from an extended family to a nuclear family and now broken families. I also believe that it is because we have sought comfort and happiness outside ourselves in material possessions, in other people and in success and we have been disappointed. I believe too that symptoms are the visible expression of invisible processes, the physical manifestations of deep emotional and sometimes spiritual difficulties, hence these symptoms must be addressed as such and not merely suppressed with drugs like tranquillisers. I believe that each of us can create a more honest way of being on this planet, for our own sakes primarily but to the benefit of everyone and everything.

3   *Weaning Yourself Off Tranquillisers*

Introduction

There are hundreds of thousands of people around the world who, through no fault of their own, find themselves faced with the problem of tranquilliser addiction. These drugs alleviate the symptoms of anxiety and can induce a sleep state but the underlying cause for the anxiety or insomnia will go untreated. The majority of people for whom tranquillisers are prescribed do not need a tranquilliser at all. Mostly they need time to express their real difficulties and a space in which to heal. Most doctors are trained to treat anxiety, insomnia, depression and other nervous disorders with pharmaceutical drugs; most do not have the time or the space to help patients with these difficulties and would therefore prefer to treat with medication or to refer the patient to a psychologist or a psychiatrist, the latter often prescribing further medicines. With the exception of acute anxiety caused by a traumatic event such as a death or serious accident, drugs have *no* role to play in the treatment of either chronic anxiety or insomnia. To treat either of these conditions with drugs has serious consequences for the patient — many of whom can't get off them — for the medical profession and for the society as a whole.

Many patients addicted to the BZs feel very guilty about being dependent on drugs, being emotionally blunted and being depressed — remember that the BZs can cause depression! Many

26

patients also feel very angry and frustrated at not having been warned in advance about the side effects of these drugs so that they could have made an informed choice. Instead they trusted their doctor.

I have visited a number of substance abuse clinics in different parts of the world and am constantly shocked by the number of doctors who end up being patients. Doctors live very stressful lives and often lose sleep or have irregular sleep patterns. Because of the easy access to drugs and because of their blind faith in pharmaceuticals, they often use drugs such as tranquillisers to help them cope. This can easily become habitual, making addiction not uncommon.

It is important to distinguish between BZ addiction and other forms of addiction. The former is more physical while addiction to heroin, morphine and alcohol is more psychological. The former results from prescribed medicine by a doctor while the latter is often self-prescribed. The former is infinitely more difficult to treat as the withdrawal effects can be severe. A number of doctors working in substance abuse clinics suggest that it is easier to get off heroin, for example, than off one of the BZs.

There is now evidence to suggest that the BZs cause not just physical dependence but psychological dependence. This evidence is based on a paper called 'BZ dependence' published in the *British Journal of Addiction* in 1981, in which Professor Malcolm Lader of the Institute of Psychiatrists in London reported that the BZs are fully capable of inducing both physical and psychological dependence.

Good Reasons to Come Off Tranquillisers
If you are addicted to one of the BZs, you may believe that it's easier to stay on the drug rather than try to come off it. However, these drugs have significant problems associated with them besides the side effects mentioned in Chapter 1.

Firstly, there are the obvious dangers associated with being drowsy, e.g. dangers driving a car, operating machinery at work, working around the home. All of these increase the risk of an accident happening.

Secondly, these drugs have a strong negative effect on one's sense of well-being. Patients on BZs often have a pale complexion and a dull or deadened facial expression, and complain of depression, lack of energy and a lack of enthusiasm for life. Relatives often complain that the patient has become irritable and moody.

Thirdly, many people have a guilt complex about not being able to get through the day without a drug; some of these people have no prior history of a nervous system disorder and may have been put on the drugs for insomnia or for trauma of whatever nature.

Fourthly, the alteration in brain chemistry as a result of taking a BZ may have serious long-term consequences. Because medical science knows so little about brain chemistry it is wiser to get off and stay off these drugs.

In 1982 at a conference at the National Institutes for Health in the USA, Professor Lader reported that the BZs when used long term can cause brain damage. He reported that brain scans done on patients who had been taking BZs for a number of years had shown a certain amount of brain damage as well as shrinkage of the brain when compared to the brains of people who had not taken BZs. Professor Lader calculated that something like one-quarter of a million patients in the UK and more than one million in the USA have taken tranquillisers for more than seven years and so could have damaged brains.

The research ties in with evidence that the BZs impair short-term memory. Research reported at a neuro-psycho-pharmacy congress in 1982 states that volunteers who have taken BZs are unable to remember things like telephone numbers, map routes, etc. There is now mounting evidence that the BZs may produce not only real physical brain damage but personality changes also. The BZs can affect your ability to enjoy life. Many patients on these drugs do not experience the normal highs and lows of life. They can alter your interaction with other people as well, especially your loved ones. If you are on one of these drugs, you may find yourself unable to relate to your spouse, your children, your relatives, your workmates, your friends, in the way you did prior to starting the drugs. Some patients on the BZs can become very aggressive. It seems a bit of a contradiction that a tranquilliser, designed to calm you, can result in aggressive behaviour.

This has been the subject of much scientific research as it stirred up a lot of controversy. In 1975 the *British Medical Journal* published an editorial entitled 'Tranquillisers causing aggression' in which the author recalled an incident where a patient taking Librium had physically assaulted his wife for the first time in their twenty years of marriage. This aggression ceased on stopping the drug. The author suggested that this aggressive behaviour was more likely to occur in people who were deeply frustrated by their home environment, work environment, interpersonal relationships, etc. On the basis of this, some doctors have suggested a link between baby battering and taking tranquillisers. Hence, doctors have to be very cautious about giving these drugs to very anxious, tense and frustrated people. BZs cannot cure anything. They can, however, hide the problem and in many instances make it worse!

Case History — David: Age Forty Years

David, a friend of mine, was put on a tranquilliser by his doctor when he discovered that his wife was having an affair with another man. He was in such emotional distress that the doctor suggested he take Valium to help him cope. He agreed but the difficulties in the marriage deepened over the next two years and they eventually separated. David stayed on the tranquilliser for this period. Once during that time he tried to come off it but got such rebound anxiety and hallucinations that he went back on it. He came to see me in desperation as he was quite frightened of trying to withdraw from it again without help.

I managed to get him off the drug in eight weeks by using a natural alternative, Nervol, which I'll speak about later in the book, and by reducing the dosage of the Valium slowly during that period. He was also able to release much of the emotional pain associated with the separation from his wife once he got off the pills. He still had difficulty dealing with stress over the following six months but after that he was emotionally and physically much stronger and able to be his old optimistic self again.

This case is very interesting as it illustrates certain problems associated with the long-term use of the BZs. Firstly, these drugs suppressed his emotions to such an extent that he was unable to feel the emotional pain associated with the breakdown of his marriage. On ceasing the drug, he was able to 'feel' again and was then able to release the tension and anger. This was a powerful growth experience for him and because of it he was able to face life again. Suppressing one's emotions with drugs is not a healing or growth experience.

Secondly, the tranquillisers caused David to be depressed to the point where he began to have a very negative view of himself and his life, which of course accentuated the difficulties he was already going through. So the drug was not only delaying his dealing with the mental problems on an emotional level, but worsening his difficulties. Thirdly, it illustrates the point that withdrawal from tranquillisers is best done with professional assistance, preferably by a doctor who has also been trained in natural medicine.

Withdrawal — Acute and Slow Withdrawal

Acute Withdrawal

Acute withdrawal is possible in a hospital environment but because it often takes place in a psychiatric ward or in a chemical dependency unit, many people prefer the option of a slow withdrawal at home. Acute withdrawal involves a six- to eight-week stay in hospital and involves substituting a long-acting BZ for a short-acting one and then slowly withdrawing the former. Other drugs are often used to control some of the severe symptoms associated with withdrawal of a BZ.

Slow withdrawal is a much wiser option and can be assisted very successfully with the use of natural medicines which I'll discuss in detail later in the book. A slow withdrawal is better as it does not require the use of further pharmaceutical drugs and gives the patient time to adjust to any underlying emotional difficulties, e.g. grief, anger.

The Open University course in the UK entitled 'Anxiety and the BZs' recommends: (a) a reduction by one-eighth of the daily dose every two to four weeks, and (b) substitution of a long-acting drug, e.g. Valium, for a short-acting one, e.g. Ativan. Again, however, it's better to do this with the help of a sympathetic doctor.

Many family doctors prefer to cut down the patient's existing dosage slowly and only if withdrawal symptoms develop do they switch from a short-acting BZ to a long-acting one. Doctors who are trained in natural medicine are much better equipped to assist a patient withdraw from tranquillisers as they have a whole battery of medicines — homoeopathic, herbal, amino acids, nutritional supplements, etc. — and therapies — hypnosis, acupuncture, etc. — to choose from. Here are some general guidelines to assist a slow withdrawal from tranquillisers, if you really want to do it alone. Later in the book I shall mention specific medicines and therapies which make withdrawal much easier.

The short-acting BZs are much more commonly prescribed as they do not cause prolonged drowsiness. Because their beneficial effect is short-lived, they need to be taken two or three times daily depending on the individual problem. Below, I have chosen to show you how to come off lorazepam (Ativan), a short-acting BZ.

Lorazepam tablets come in 1 mg (blue) and 2.5 mg (yellow) tablets. These tablets may be difficult to cut in half but often your pharmacist will help by doing this for you.

If you are on, say, three 1 mg tablets daily cut this down immediately to 2.5 mg. Table 3.1 explains the withdrawal procedure in detail.

Table 3.1 Getting off lorazepam (Ativan)

	Morning	Afternoon	Evening	Total daily dose
Prescribed dose:	1 mg	1 mg	1 mg	(3 mg)
Immediately	1 mg	½ mg	1 mg	(2½ mg)
One month later	1 mg	½ mg	½ mg	(2 mg)
One month later	½ mg	½ mg	½ mg	(1½ mg)
One month later	½ mg	–	½ mg	(1 mg)
One month later	½ mg	–	–	(½ mg)
One month later	0 mg	–	–	(0 mg)
Well done!				

This slow method of withdrawal takes five months in all. In many patients this can be reduced to two and a half to three months with the use of natural medicines. It is important to understand that even after coming off the drugs, there will still be a recovery period where your body's chemistry, your REM sleep pattern and your emotions must return to normal. This period can vary from six months to two years depending on the individual patient and on how long he/she has been on the tranquilliser.

Making Withdrawal Easier

I shall discuss how to use a range of medicines, including herbals, homoeopathics and nutritional supplements, under those chapter headings later in the book. However, there is a particular therapy which I cannot fail to mention and since it will not be discussed elsewhere in the book, let's discuss it now. I am speaking about acupuncture.

In making withdrawal easier and virtually side-effect-free, acupuncture ranks as the single most successful therapy. Ear acupuncture (auriculo-therapy) is the treatment of choice in helping drug addicts not just to get off but to stay off a whole range of licit and illicit drugs.

In 1989 the *Lancet*, a respected medical journal, documented a study noting that when acupuncture was added to the treatment of chronic alcoholics, the percentage of those completing the programme successfully increased significantly. Furthermore, it reduced their craving for alcohol, with much fewer relapses. Other studies have illustrated the success of acupuncture in the treatment of opium and heroin addictions, with a 100 per cent success rate in alleviating the symptoms of withdrawal.

Dr Jay Holder, director of a residential treatment hospital for addicts in Miami, has developed a form of auriculo-therapy for addiction treatment. He reports success rates of over 80 per cent for nicotine, alcohol, cocaine, heroin and BZ addicts. For his work, Dr Holder was the first American doctor to be awarded the Albert Schweitzer prize in medicine. Today there are 300 treatment centres in the USA using acupuncture to treat substance abuse. Because of the amazing success of these treatment centres, similar centres have been established in many other countries, including Canada, Mexico, the UK, Sweden, Germany and Spain. What is interesting is that the medical profession has been slow to accept this form of treatment despite its obvious success. However, the legal profession, especially judges who are faced with drug addicts every day, have accepted the idea of acupuncture and are referring addicts for treatment rather than sending them to jail. Drug addiction is after all a medical problem not a legal one!

Acupuncture is not only effective for drug withdrawal symptoms but according to Professor Pierre Huard of the Medical Faculty of Paris, it 'is equivalent to the effect of tranquillisers in cases of depression, anxiety, insomnia and nervous disorders and its action is swift and lasting'.

The US House of Representatives and the Senate

Appropriations Committee have voted in favour of acupuncture for substance abuse recovery as it is extremely cost-effective.

All in all, acupuncture is the single most important treatment not just for BZ withdrawal but for alcohol, tobacco, heroin and opiate withdrawal and for many other forms of addiction including work, sex and gambling addictions and food disorders. Acupuncture is also very successful as a non-drug form of treatment for anxiety, depression and insomnia. If you wish to use acupuncture to ease your withdrawal from a tranquilliser or you just want treatment for a nervous disorder, go to an acupuncturist trained in ear acupuncture as this form is particularly successful.

Summary

There are thousands of people around the world who through no fault of their own are faced with the problem of tranquilliser addiction. If you are one of these people and you would like to get off the tranquilliser it is best to do this with professional help. There is a fast method of withdrawal, usually done only in hospital or a chemical dependency unit, or a slow way which can be done at home with professional assistance. If you experience side effects, these are best treated with natural medicines or with natural therapies such as acupuncture. Acupuncture has achieved worldwide fame not just for the treatment of various forms of addiction but for helping nervous conditions such as depression, anxiety and insomnia.

Viewing the Patient
4   *with Different Eyes*

Introduction

Day after day I see people in my surgery with a variety of physical symptoms — bowel disturbances, palpitations, excessive sweating, heart arrhythmias, headaches, insomnia, etc. — which do not originate in the physical body. Many of these people think that their illness has struck them by some quirk of Nature; they do not see their role in the development of this illness as it is easier to believe that it comes from outside them — work stress, bad marital relationships, pressure of time, financial problems. The truth is rather different and more difficult to accept. All illness originates deep inside you; you are the designer, originator, creator of your own sickness. The physical expression of this illness or sickness serves the purpose of reminding you of the deeper, often emotional, source of the disease. Treating the physical symptoms and signs of the illness helps temporarily to bury the emotional or deeper aspects but as sure as the grass is green the illness will resurface at some future point in time. It is all too easy to believe that the symptoms and signs are physical in origin and can be treated as such, and the relief with modern drugs is so quick that it supports this belief system. There are two ways of viewing everything — indeed many ways!

Two Sides to Everything

If you, the reader, are viewing the back of my hand you will see

35

nails on the tops of my fingers and hairs on the fingers and lower down on the hand and wrist. However, if I am viewing the other side of my hand, i.e. the palm, I won't be able to see any nails or hairs; I shall see bare skin. Hence, there are two ways of viewing the same hand. We are each seeing one side of the story but are unable to see both sides simultaneously; hence, the difficulty you might have in believing in what I'm telling you about my hand and vice versa. Being able to see both sides at once and accepting the importance of both sides is the key to understanding the physical and metaphysical aspects of ourselves.

The human being has many levels of expression but for the sake of simplicity I shall describe four of them.

An easy way of understanding the different levels of a human being is to revise one's knowledge of basic science. At school you may have learned about the molecular structure of solids, liquids and gases. Solids are made up of molecules densely packed together which vibrate at a low frequency or energy, in liquids the molecules are less densely packed and vibrate at a higher frequency, while in gases the molecules are of very high frequency and energy and have no density, i.e. the molecules float around and have little or no form or shape.

Figure 4.1

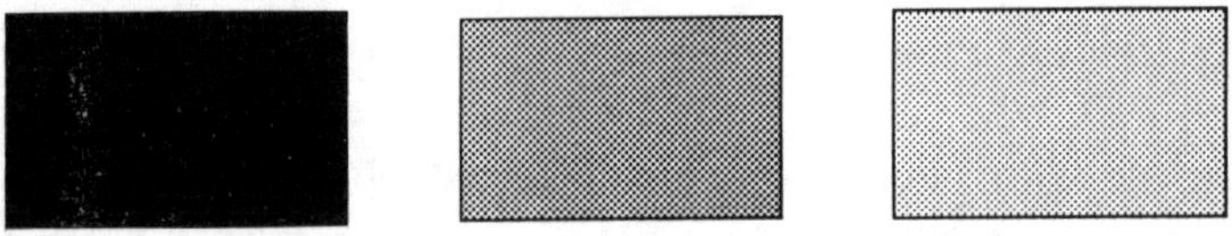

Solid	Liquid	Gas
Molecules densely packed	Molecules further apart	Molecules far apart
Molecules of low energy	Molecules have higher energy	Molecules vibrate at very high energy
Solids have shape or form	Liquids take on the shape of the vessel that they are in	
(Shape or form)	(Shapeless) but visible	Mostly invisible

In Figure 4.1, you can see that matter is really condensed energy, i.e. molecules densely packed together. The more densely packed they are, the more dense or physical the structure will be.

If you now regard the physical body of a human as a solid structure of low vibrational energy and the soul as a gas of very high energy which is invisible to most people and the mental and emotional bodies in between these two, you get a reasonable idea of what I mean by the different levels that make up a human being. The physical body is more dense and so has form or shape that you can see. Often this form or shape is a reflection of the energy of one's soul. The spiritual body lacks density or form and because it can float, in the same way that gases do, it can leave the physical body as in a near-death experience or as death itself. The emotional body is of a lower energy than the spiritual body, and the mental body or mind lower still. These four levels of one's being are represented graphically in Figure 4.2.

Figure 4.2

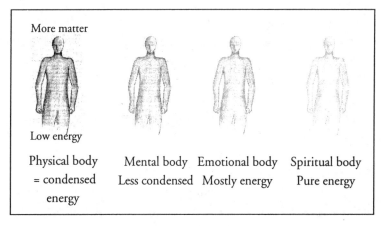

More matter

Low energy

Physical body = condensed energy | Mental body Less condensed | Emotional body Mostly energy | Spiritual body Pure energy

One's experiences in life have the power to uplift the soul, i.e. increase the vibrational energy, making it more subtle or nebulous, but may also have the power to depress the soul's energy, making it of a lower energy. People who live their lives from a base of fear often have a lower spiritual energy and will therefore have a negative or depressing effect on others. People who live their lives from a base of love often have a high vibrational energy which uplifts others.

The Spiritual Body

The core of your being, the real you, the light deep within is your soul or spiritual body. It needs love in the same way that your physical body needs food. The receipt of love as a child makes us spiritually stronger and this love connects you with others (your parents, siblings, relatives, friends) and with the rest of Nature. Fear is the absence of love. Fear is nothing of itself, merely the absence of something, in the same way that darkness is nothing other than the absence of light. Yet, for most people in the Western world fear dominates and rules our lives — fear of death, fear of not having enough, fear of failure, fear, fear, fear! This is the root cause of most human illness. Why is this so? I believe that we have lost touch with our souls, with our true selves and are unable to love unconditionally. Out of fear we need to control and even the love we express is of a controlling nature, i.e. conditional. It is not given freely and innocently, i.e. selflessly. It's given only if we receive something in return. Your soul is like an old-fashioned paraffin lamp in that love will make it glow brightly while little or no love will reduce the flame and may extinguish it completely. We are beings of love; in fact, the whole of creation is energised by love. This is why many religions speak of God and love as one and the same.

The Emotional Body

Next I wish to speak of the emotional body. In terms of illness, this is the most important place to go looking for problems. In the Western world we are physically and mentally very active, running around chasing our tails with our heads full of things to remember to do, almost to the point of being very inactive emotionally. We have little time to feel, to listen to our hearts, let alone express those feelings. Functioning physically and mentally and blocking our emotions is a more comfortable and more convenient way to exist. However, life is about love, not comfort and convenience, and love acts from the spirit or soul of the person through the emotional or feeling body. To block this emotional or feeling body is to block one's very essence, i.e. you suffocate your true self. By doing so you have an unseen negative effect on the souls of others. People are uplifted by a free, loving, innocent soul and 'downlifted' by a false, blocked, unloving, unemotional soul. Your energy interacts with and affects everyone around you. I feel very sad when I see someone who is blocked emotionally, especially when they are unable to acknowledge it. Emotional blockages are the biggest threat to your health and well-being. Blocked anger is particularly dangerous.

Case History — Brenda: Age Thirty-Eight Years

Brenda had suffered from bowel problems continuously for eight years and as she was getting worse — to the point where she was becoming intolerant to many of the foods which had previously formed the bulk of her diet — she began to seek help. After eating wheat, dairy produce, sugary foods, yeast foods and potatoes she developed abdominal bloating, loose, pale, offensive stool, flatulence, and a significant drop in her energy level. She also suffered from hypoglycaemia (low blood sugar levels) occasionally, cold peripheries and irritability. I diagnosed her as suffering from pancreatitis, a condition that is common but is seldom diagnosed. I treated her using *chromium picolinate*, high-potency B complex, pancreatic enzymes and a homoeopathic medicine, *momordica balsamina*, in high potency, and used a restricted diet. Because chronic pancreatitis is often a manifestation of internalised stress, we discussed the sources of stress in her life. To cut a long story short, she had a tremendous anger directed against her father, who was alcoholic and had abandoned the family when Brenda was nine years old. Since the upper abdomen is an emotional zone in the body, deep-felt emotions such as anger manifest in this region, sometimes affecting the pancreas as was the case with Brenda. Today she is physically and emotionally much stronger and is now able to tolerate a normal diet. In Brenda's case it was necessary to treat her both physically and emotionally simultaneously to gain this improvement.

The Spiritual Body or Soul — Further Notes
There are only two energies that affect the soul — love and fear. Love is a positive energy that has an uplifting effect on all levels of one's being; it makes you glow brightly. Love is the core of a human being; it is not just nourishment for the soul but a radiance that reaches through to the physical and illuminates it. Love is what every human being craves. It is the foundation of a child's life. Children are beings of love and light and they need constant reassurance on a daily basis that they are loved. When they get it they feel secure and it strengthens them inwardly to enable them to deal with life's difficulties. Where this love is absent or deficient, fear enters the picture.

Fear, or the absence of love, has a negative effect on all levels of one's being. It makes whatever light radiates from your soul shrink. It weakens the human spirit and is often used by parents, priests, teachers, doctors, lawyers and other people and structures in the society to control your spirit. Fear cuts you off from love as the two energies are diametrically opposed to one another, i.e. you cannot experience love while in a state of fear and vice versa.

I lived for two years in West Africa, where children are born into an extended family and where the child experiences love and warmth not just from its parents but from its grandparents, aunts and uncles and so on, all of whom live close to one another. Babies are carried on the mother's back and are breastfed for the first two to three years of life; this close physical contact with the mother has a strengthening effect emotionally and spiritually. The human warmth exuded by those people is a shock for us Westerners, even the Irish, who are regarded as particularly warm and friendly. By comparison our society is much colder, the family unit is often fragmented into a nuclear or single-parent family and the physical bonding between mother and child often minimal, especially if the mother works, which is fast becoming the norm.

Western society is all about money and — the word that I have great difficulty with — 'progress'. If building concrete jungles, destroying Nature and people who live according to Nature, destroying the family bonds, especially between mother and baby, and putting people under more and more stress to make more money so that they can survive (not live peacefully) is called progress, then one must question the meaning of this word.

In addition, our society is about greed and power and control. We give away our individual power to politicians, allowing them carte blanche to do what they wish, and many seem to be able to get away with blatant corruption; we call this process democracy but it has little to do with democracy. In a democratic process people retain their power and vote on important issues affecting their lives; in our system of government money from companies and organisations with powerful political lobbies controls to a great extent what happens to the rest of us. Obviously this process is changing and the youth in Europe are no longer accepting the power and control of the major structures in the society. For example, the Catholic church in Ireland had a strong influence on Irish politics for many years. Because the church is so wealthy and so powerful it can exert its influence on many aspects of the life of an average Irish person. Today, the youth are no longer attending church in the way their parents did, nor are they giving blind respect to an organisation that is clearly out of touch with their needs. The church that influenced my life growing up in Ireland used fear as the means to control; if you didn't attend church God would punish you. I don't see how a loving God can punish you for not agreeing with him. If one is working from a base of love and compassion, one's aim is to understand and help the person, not to punish.

Fear controls one's spirit; love sets you free. The route to freeing your soul is to live your life as you see fit and not in accordance with the rules set down by your parents, teachers or society. These rules are often based in negativity and fear which deplete your spiritual energy. The aim for each of us in life is simply to 'be oneself'.

Rose was one person who had enormous difficulty acknowledging her own needs. She had a very mundane job in an insurance company but in her spare time she used to write poetry. She came to me because she had high blood pressure, a fast heart rate, and palpitations. It took some time to get her blood pressure under control; it took an even longer time to get her to open up emotionally and speak about her feelings. One day I asked to see some of her poems and when I read them I saw the reason for her difficulties and why it took so long for her physical symptoms to improve. Her poems described a person locked deep inside, almost to the point of suffocation, who was crying out for love. Her soul spoke through these poems but otherwise was being kept silent. She was finding it more and more difficult to stop her heart from expressing itself and this led to conflict as she was frightened to allow it full expression. She was unmarried and had never had an intimate loving relationship with anyone.

Through being encouraged to trust her feelings and to trust in other people, she began to change and over a period of time it became easier and easier to keep her physical symptoms under control. Today she is still on low-dose medication but is working hard at changing her old patterns of behaviour — she rang me recently to tell me that she was changing her job and leaving the insurance company. I was delighted to hear this as it represented a move away from security and taking a step into the unknown.

Mental Body or Mind
This is the part of your being from where thoughts emanate. These thoughts can uplift, comfort and please you or they can have the opposite effect, i.e. create disharmony, upset and keep you trapped in a particular mode of behaviour. Since thought precedes action, the mind has a powerful controlling influence on the physical body. A sustained pattern of positive thinking can maintain harmony and so good health in the physical body; a sustained pattern of negative thinking will inevitably result in

physical disharmony or ill health. The proponents of positive thinking therefore are absolutely right since positive thoughts do reflect in the physical body as better health as well as a better attitude in our dealings with others, in our work and in our environment in general.

How you think about yourself is critical to your ability to develop your own potential as a human being. If you think highly of yourself and are aware of your own abilities, you will achieve the goals that you set for yourself. In the Western world, however, so many people have such low self-esteem. This lack of self-belief guarantees failure in almost anything you try. The way to reverse this pattern of negative thinking is quite simple, as most people in the world of advertising know. You simply repeat positive messages over and over, whether mentally or by reading them or by saying them out loud. Advertisers know that if you repeat the same message day after day, you will begin to believe it, no matter how ridiculous the message may seem. Companies spend large sums of money on advertising because it works. Your mind or thoughts can be influenced. You can use this fact in a therapeutic sense. Simply repeat a series of positive messages daily and you will begin to believe them and then you will begin to act in a positive way. How you feel about yourself is at the very heart of all self-improvement. For people with low self-esteem here is a series of positive messages for you to read or say out loud morning and evening:

I am lovable, worthwhile and capable.
I am a special person.
I exude self-confidence and personal power.
I love the world and the world loves me.
I deserve the very best in life.
I am willing to be happy and successful.
I accept myself completely here and now.
I am strong and secure.
I am more and more in charge of my life.
Who I am makes a difference.
I choose my response.

43

Healing the Energy of the Patient

To help a patient, I first have to recognise where the major disturbance is in the person — it's usually in the emotional body as repressed anger or in the spiritual body as fear. I then have to assist the physical body whether or not the patient recognises the source of the disturbance. Because the patient usually presents with physical symptoms it is important to assist at this level but also to subtly or in some cases blatantly assist at other levels.

How the Different Levels of One's Being Interact

If fear is the dominant energy affecting one's soul, this will alter the energy of the emotional body in a negative way and cause anxiety, which in turn will set a negative thought pattern in the mind, which in turn will precipitate physical symptoms over which the patient feels they have little or no control. This is why I often make the statement that fear is the root cause of most illness. This interaction between our different bodies, or energy levels, is illustrated graphically below. Because the soul's energy is of such a high level, its energy envelopes and interacts with all the other bodies. The circles below should really overlap one another. The aim of healing is to increase the energy of one's soul, which will automatically have a positive knock-on effect on everything else, especially one's physical symptoms. Healers themselves must have a high spiritual energy, or high level of self-awareness, and must have the tools with which to alter a patient's energy.

Figure 4.3

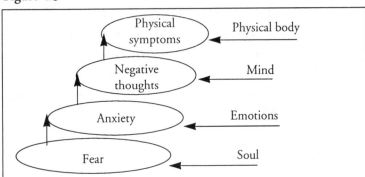

As you can see from this, healing is a complicated business and yet desperately simple in another sense. The source of human illness, especially in Western society, is simple to understand, but it can be complicated to find the exact medicines and techniques to bring about a healing in the person to the point where recurrence is unlikely.

This is especially so for people on tranquillisers as they are often dulled mentally and emotionally, i.e. of reduced energy at these levels, and are often frightened of coming off these drugs and in some cases of dealing with the reason why they were put on them in the first instance — e.g. trauma, rape, relationship break-up, death of a loved one and so on. Many people who are on tranquillisers are on an antidepressant at the same time, making withdrawal and increasing their energy levels that bit more complex. In helping such patients it is often necessary to work with all levels of their being concomitantly. This can involve the following:

- weaning them off the tranquillisers and/or antidepressants
- using a natural tranquilliser and/or antidepressant
- encouraging positive mental thought patterns
- allowing space and time for emotional pain to be released
- encouraging relaxation, meditation and visualisation techniques

Summary

In essence then it is essential to view physical symptoms in a wider context and never to take them at face value, as you can miss so much. Seeing in behind the physical symptoms is like seeing the magic of life and the magic of human beings at work — it is fascinating to view the insides of people's lives! I never get bored in my work as each person's life is like a piece of a jigsaw puzzle which becomes clearer and clearer. By reflecting back to the patient what I can see happening in his/her life, I hope I am able to provide insights he/she may not have had before. Through this insight the patient is able to see himself or herself in a different way; this is often the first step towards change.

5 *Hypnosis*

Hypnosis is no stranger to you. It is really the state you enter before you fall asleep; that in-between state where you are neither fully asleep nor fully awake; that pleasant, relaxed, almost immobilised state where you are physically and mentally switched off yet aware of what is going on around you. It is a beautiful, peaceful state where movement and thoughts come to rest, where a pleasant wave of relaxation passes through you. You can enter the sleep state very easily and you can also enter the awakened state very easily from this hypnotic or trance state.

When physical activity and mental thoughts are brought to rest, it is possible to hear and experience the deeper side of yourself, to gain a deeper understanding of some of the dynamics that make you tick as a person. Your inner world becomes more accessible and you gain a greater understanding of why you think the way you do and why you behave the way you do. With this greater understanding, you are then able to change the way you *feel* and hence the way you *think* and *act*.

A Personal Note

For many years I felt bad about myself, pulling myself down every chance I got. I was very self-centred and as a consequence very critical of everyone and everything around me. I graduated from two universities (one of them Trinity College, Dublin, one of the most famous universities in the world), with a science degree from one and a medical degree from the other and yet did not go to either graduation ceremony. I didn't understand this behaviour, nor my high level of self-criticism, until a stranger came into my surgery in Dublin one day. It was autumn in Ireland and was cold and wet and windy. I had just finished work when my receptionist told me that there was a therapist from Australia visiting Dublin who would like to speak with me for a few minutes. I called him in. He was dressed in a long brown trenchcoat with a wide-brimmed hat; he had obviously come to Ireland prepared for bad weather! We spoke for about thirty minutes, during which time he told me that he had been trained as a hypnotherapist in New South Wales, and after having been in Australia for twenty years he wanted to come back to Ireland, where he had lived as a child.

During the conversation it became apparent to me that not only would we work well together but it was as if I knew him even though our paths had not crossed before. He stayed in Ireland working with me for some time and he became a great teacher and a great friend, helping me to gain enormous insight into why I was so negative and so self-critical. It was a turning point in my life and I wish to thank him again for his help in changing me. They say that the teacher arrives when the student is ready and this was clearly the case in my life. I was searching for a deeper understanding of myself and wanted to stop repeating patterns of downplaying myself all the time. He taught me how powerful hypnosis can be in facilitating change in one's life. A lot of my difficulty centred on my father, who was absent for most of my life, through no fault of his own. When he came home, usually at Easter and Christmas, he was unable to show any love or affection for me and was often very harshly critical. At various points while growing up, I needed him for emotional and spiritual support and needed him to tell me I was doing fine. Although I was a talented athlete and footballer, and quite intelligent, I never achieved my potential simply because I didn't believe myself worthy of success. Hypnosis was enormously helpful to me in that it gave me a clear understanding of why I had such low self-esteem but it also helped reprogramme my subconscious mind to boost my self-confidence and allow me for the first time really to believe in myself. It was an enormously uplifting experience and I am now able to practise self-hypnosis on a regular basis.

Self-hypnosis is simply getting oneself into a relaxed state (the subconscious mind is more receptive in this state) and playing a tape with positive messages on it. If you do this daily or better still first thing in the morning and last thing at night, your mind will begin to accept those positive statements as real and hence negative thought patterns will change and become more positive, and emotionally your anxiety will dissipate and you will feel more at ease. Self-hypnosis 'works', as many advertisers know well. Some of the major companies spend millions of dollars advertising their soft drink or washing powder or whatever. They know that if you hear a message repeatedly it will eventually sink in and have the desired effect. Self-hypnosis is one of the most powerful healing tools available and accessible to you.

Writing down positive statements, or affirmations, and reading them daily is an alternative way of doing this. Because one is often reading them in a more alert, non-relaxed state, they do not have as deep or as powerful an effect; the more relaxed you are, the more open your subconscious mind is to suggestions. However, affirmations are helpful and I would recommend that you read these positive statements provided you use your own words and you phrase the statement in a positive way, e.g. 'I interpret everything that happens to me in a positive way,' instead of 'I interpret everything that happens to me in a less negative way.'

The History of Hypnosis
Entering into a trance state is one of the oldest forms of healing. The native American Indians dance in a circular fashion around a lighted fire to the sound of drums beating out a repetitive rhythm. The repetitive movement in a circle to a background musical rhythm dulls the physical and mental activity and leads to a trance state being induced naturally or spontaneously.

The tribes that I lived with in West Africa used to perform

healing ceremonies in a similar fashion. The Bushmen of Southern Africa do likewise.

Old medical textbooks held that healing which occurred in the trance state was divinely inspired and that the miraculous cures which often resulted were spiritual in nature. In ancient Greece one of the classical methods of healing involved travelling long distances to one of the shrines such as the Temple of Aesculapius at Epidaurus, which contained a statue believed to be endowed with miraculous powers. The patients, after their long and tiring journeys, would present offerings at the gates of the Temple. They would then spend a few days and nights praying in the surroundings and only after a period of time would be admitted to the Temple itself. Inside, help was given by laying on of hands, by oracles or in the form of prophetic dreams. This air of mysticism, ceremony and ritual was highly important, as in the case of the Bushmen and others, as it produced an air of expectancy in people whose belief was strong.

Entering the Hypnotic State

In 1953 Bernard Gindes suggested in his book *New Concepts of Hypnosis* that for a person to enter the hypnotic state their *attention* must be focused; they must *believe* that it will work; and the ceremony/ritual aspect adds the final ingredient, i.e. the air of *expectation* that something magical or mystical can occur.

ATTENTION AND BELIEF AND EXPECTATION = THE HYPNOTIC STATE

In modern times, the statue of Our Lady at Lourdes, France serves a similar function to the temples of ancient Greece. Thousands come from all over the world who *believe* in the healing power of the statue, to a place — Lourdes — where miracle cures have occurred in the past and can be *expected* to occur again. One's *attention* is focused via various rituals and ceremonies, paving the way for a trance or hypnotic state on entering the grotto. In this hypnotic state, healing can indeed take place.

The Father of Modern Hypnosis

Dr August Liébeault from France is considered to be the father of modern hypnosis. In the late 1800s Dr Liébeault was a country doctor near Nancy, who became fascinated by the power of hypnosis in treating various ailments. He was the first to illustrate the curative value of hypnosis on a large scale, having successfully treated thousands of patients.

His work attracted the attention of a famous neurologist, Professor Hippolyte-Marie Bernheim. Bernheim was so impressed with Dr Liébeault's work that he went on to promote the benefits of hypnosis and rapidly became one of the greatest authorities on the subject. Such was Bernheim's reputation that the medical profession was forced to recognise the power of hypnosis to heal.

These two Frenchmen did much to bring hypnosis out of the occult and into acceptable medical practice. Through their successes, hypnosis gained significant acceptability throughout Europe, so laying the foundation for its use today. They showed that entering the hypnotic state was a natural, spontaneous phenomenon, if the right conditions were provided. They gave hypnosis respectability.

A Patient Called Bertha

In 1881 Bertha Pappenheim, the 21-year-old daughter of a Viennese grain merchant, sought treatment from a Dr Josef Brewer in Vienna. Bertha had nursed her father for several months prior to his death in April of that year. As a result, her health had deteriorated and she developed rather unusual symptoms — cough, visual disturbance, paralysis, visions of snakes. Because of the nature of her symptoms, Dr Brewer decided to use hypnosis to help her.

While in the hypnotic state, the young girl regressed spontaneously and began to talk of her experiences and problems, culminating in a profound emotional release which was followed by the disappearance of many of her symptoms. Her case was very interesting in that it was the first time that a patient had regressed and begun to speak spontaneously under hypnosis. Bertha also illustrated another important point, i.e. her profound emotional release while under hypnosis led to the disappearance of many of her physical symptoms. In other words, hypnosis had treated the underlying cause of her symptoms; this cause was clearly emotional in nature and had been repressed, which in turn led to the development of her physical symptoms.

The fact that hypnosis was shown to be effective in treating the underlying cause of Bertha's symptoms further validated the potential of hypnosis in healing human illness.

Desensitisation
Despite its obvious effectiveness, the medical profession still did not embrace hypnosis, favouring chemical drugs as the main form of treating human ailments. This attitude persists today, excluding a small number of doctors and dentists who have become convinced of the power of hypnosis and use it in their individual practices.

In 1958 Joseph Wolfe took hypnosis a step further by developing a form of treatment known as desensitisation. This means that a person can be 'desensitised' to an event or place that they interpret as frightening or threatening. For example, if you have a fear of flying, it is possible to 'desensitise' you under hypnosis and to recondition your mind to interpret the act of flying as pleasant and enjoyable. Treatment by desensitisation under hypnosis is well described in Wolfe's book *Psychotherapy by Reciprocal Inhibition* (Stanford University Press: 1958) and this has now become an established form of treatment for a range of phobias — further evidence of the benefits of hypnosis.

Hypnosis and the Medical Establishment
Despite the fact that hypnosis is ancient in its origins and has been used as the main form of healing by many cultures around the globe, and despite the fact that many medical doctors have demonstrated its enormous therapeutic benefits, it remains a 'fringe' form of medical treatment. In most medical and dental schools around the world it is not taught to students.

In 1953 the Psychological Medicine Group Committee of the British Medical Association appointed a subcommittee to consider the use of hypnosis. Its report, published in 1955, recommended that basic lectures be given to medical undergraduates and clinical instruction be given to postgraduate students in the fields of psychiatry, anaesthesiology and obstetrics. However, to this day this advice has been largely ignored.

Uses of Hypnosis

1. NERVOUS DISORDERS
Hypnosis must be the treatment of choice in a range of nervous disorders including anxiety, phobias, obsessive-compulsive disorder, and psychosomatic illness.

2. NERVOUS HABITS
Habits such as blushing, muscle spasms, tics, stammering, nail-biting, etc. are also relatively easy to treat using hypnosis.

3. CHEMICAL DEPENDENCE
Because of its ability to access emotional pain, hypnosis can often be very helpful in the treatment of alcoholism and drug addiction as well as smoking. It is also extremely helpful in treating eating disorders such as anorexia and bulimia, for the same reason.

4. SEXUAL PROBLEMS
A range of sexual problems in males and females can be treated effectively using hypnosis. These problems range from impotence and premature ejaculation in men to vaginismus and frigidity in females to loss of libido and absence of orgasm in both sexes.

5. OTHER PROBLEMS
Because of its ability to alleviate pain, hypnosis is often used by dentists, by obstetricians at childbirth and by surgeons. The cancer surgeon and author Bernie Segal often uses it while operating on his patients to alleviate post-operative pain and to accelerate healing of the tissues.

Hypnosis is particularly relevant in the treatment of terminally ill patients to alleviate pain and to facilitate a more dignified death.

Personally, I have found hypnosis to be most beneficial in (a) giving people an understanding of why they are repeating certain patterns of behaviour in their lives, e.g. attracting the same type of boyfriend/girlfriend, (b) removing fears and phobias which are the main obstacle to human health and happiness, and (c) boosting a person's self-esteem, making them more aware of the beauty and love within each of us. As you can see, hypnosis can be a powerful tool in human growth.

Conditions in which Hypnosis Should Not Be Used

1. PSYCHIATRIC DISORDERS
These include depression, schizophrenia, psychosis, mentally subnormal patients.

2. PHYSICAL DISORDERS
These include thyroid dysfunction, hypoglycaemia (low blood sugar level) and brain tumours.

3. OTHER SITUATIONS
Hypnosis should never be used if the patient objects to treatment. I find that many patients, particularly in South Africa, have a fear of hypnosis. Hypnosis should not be repeated if the patient has had a significant reaction in a negative sense to the first or second treatment. I have had one patient who had an out-of-body experience after her first treatment. It took quite a long time for her to stabilise again after this. Because her reaction was somewhat severe and unique, I decided not to repeat hypnosis with her.

Generally, hypnosis is a wonderful therapy but it should be used only where it is clinically applicable, and continued where the patient is clearly benefiting.

I find that hypnosis can be combined wonderfully with creative visualisation provided the patient is capable of visualising. Creative visualisation allows the patient to create a mental picture of what he/she wishes for and to live as if this picture were real, feeling and experiencing the positive benefits of it at that moment.

Do not be frightened of hypnosis. It is a beautiful relaxed state in which magical things can happen for your upliftment as a human being. If you would like to know more about hypnosis read books on the therapeutic benefits of hypnosis or visit a clinical hypnotherapist and he/she can assess if hypnosis would be of benefit to you. It has the power to transform your life.

Case History — Mary: Age Forty-Five Years

Mary was a nun in a convent in a small town outside of Dublin and came to me because she had a problem with blushing in the presence of others. She was a very shy and timid person with a high anxiety level. She found that the problem was particularly acute when she attended choir practice each morning before breakfast.

I used hypnosis to assist her by getting her deeply relaxed and desensitising her to anxiety-producing situations, e.g. choir practice, then using ego-strengthening techniques to improve her self-image. I also made a self-hypnosis tape for her to use daily in the convent. After five sessions she found that the blushing had decreased a lot. By the eighth session, it was gone completely and her self-esteem had increased considerably. In addition, she used a herb called kava kava for a period of three months and is now much more relaxed in the presence of others.

Summary
Hypnosis is a state of deep relaxation in which you are still aware of your surroundings. In this state, your subconscious mind is more open to suggestion, so making it possible to reprogramme this part of the mind in a positive way by suggesting feelings of well-being, calmness and so on. Because hypnosis helps make your inner world more accessible, it is possible to remove the greatest blocks to much human health and happiness, i.e. fears or phobias of all sorts. One is also able to gain an understanding of

why we repeat certain patterns of behaviour in our lives, e.g. comfort eating. With this understanding you are then able to make fundamental or profound changes in your life in the way you feel and hence in the way you think and act.

Hypnosis can, through reducing the power of negativity and increasing our power to be positive, lead to tremendous self-development, and personally I would regard it as the single most important tool to accelerate or speed up one's self-awareness or growth as a human being.

6   *Herbal Medicine*

Herbal medicine is the oldest and most tried and tested form of medicine. In a sense it is degrading to refer to it as an 'alternative', since it forms the basis of all medicine — conventional drugs, homoeopathic medicine, traditional Chinese medicines, etc. It is the original medicine, the mother of all remedies used today. Herbal medicine has been used by all cultures for centuries and is still the main form of medical treatment among 80 per cent of the world's population. It is sad to hear some doctors describing herbal medicine as quackery since many of today's drugs (e.g. quinine, reserpine, ephedrine, ipecac) come directly from plants, while most synthetic drugs are based on chemicals extracted from herbs. Why has the medical profession not embraced herbal medicines in the same way that it has synthetically produced drugs? I believe the answer has to do with money and power, although teaching methods in medical schools are also a factor.

First of all, there is no big money in herbs. Herbal medicines cannot be patented so there is no incentive to produce them on a large scale. Drugs, regardless of whether they are produced synthetically or isolated from herbal extracts, can be patented, bottled and sold for incredible sums of money. This is what pharmaceutical companies do. This is why they are so wealthy and capable of financing many medical projects.

The way in which doctors are educated at medical school is another reason why herbal medicine has not been embraced by the medical profession. Medical education is not holistic. It makes no attempt to deal with people on anything other than a physical level. The main form of treatment, even when dealing with sensitive emotional issues, is pharmaceutical drugs. No attempt is made to educate doctors on issues as fundamental as nutrition. You only have to look at the food served in hospital canteens and coffee shops to see the incredible lack of awareness among doctors in this regard — ironically it is often their job to treat people with nutritional imbalances.

Herbal medicine and nutrition must form the cornerstone of medical therapeutics if people are to be *healed* as distinct from *treated*. At present, the only form of therapeutics taught to medical students in university is pharmacology — the study and use of chemical drugs. The medical profession must choose between money and power on the one hand and the good of humanity on the other. When next you see negative reports in the media about herbal medicine, remember that this is the most important form of medicine for the majority of people on the planet, especially those who cannot afford expensive drugs.

Herbs — Part of Nature's Energy Cycle

All life on this planet depends on the sun. The sun provides us with light and heat energy. Plants use light energy to make food in an amazing process called photosynthesis. This process converts energy into matter (food). In addition to being vital for our survival, photosynthesis beautifully exemplifies one of Albert Einstein's theories — that energy and matter are the same thing, and that one can be converted into the other.

While photosynthesis shows how energy can be converted into matter, there is another remarkable process which can convert matter (food) back into energy. This process is called respiration. When we eat the food in a plant, it is broken down into smaller units (digested) and eventually ends up being used in respiration to provide energy for the body. Many forms of alternative medicine use both matter (a herb, for example) and energy (e.g. homoeopathic medicine) to heal people. Scientists who have difficulty in understanding how energy-based medicine such as homoeopathy and acupuncture work need only revise basic biology and physics.

Figure 6.1

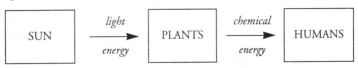

Figure 6.1 illustrates an important point — when you use herbs or plants for healing you are part of an energy transfer and, therefore, part of Nature. This energy is universal (from the sun in this example) and flows through Nature to you. By using the herb, you are actually part of something much greater — you are linked into something happening millions of miles from earth. This is why natural medicines are so wonderful to use — they work at different levels within you, not just the physical.

Herbal Medicines and Synthetic Drugs: A Comparison
In 1874, sodium salicylate (synthetic aspirin) was synthesised chemically in a laboratory for the first time. This led to a surge in the use of synthetic medicines and a decline in the use of herbs. We assumed that all our medicines could be produced in laboratories and that Nature would become redundant. Gradually, however, this assumption has been dispelled. The thalidomide disaster in the 1950s was a major warning sign of the danger of using synthetically produced medicines. In the 1980s, Opren — an anti-inflammatory drug used to treat arthritis — killed a number of patients suffering from that condition. In June 1986, all children's medicine containing aspirin had to be taken off the market because a number of children had died from brain and liver damage (Reye's Syndrome). The problem of side effects has weakened considerably the arguments in favour of using synthetic drugs. Today, most people are justifiably concerned about the use of conventional medicines.

Not all aspects of chemical analysis and laboratory research are negative, though. In fact, the scientific knowledge we have gained has been of considerable value. It has, for example, proven beyond doubt the claims made by ancient healers about certain plants. The shamans (traditional doctors) of the North American Indians have claimed that plants such as *Echinacea purpurea* and *Baptisia tinctoria* can be used to treat infections. Scientific researchers have isolated particular chemicals (called glycoproteins and polysaccharides) from these herbs and found that they stimulate the immune system as well as damaging invading bacteria. Hence, modern techniques have substantiated what 'primitive' healers have been saying for some time — that these herbs are effective in the treatment of infections.

Scientists have also analysed a herb called Meadowsweet (*Filipendula ulmaria*) and found that it contains a natural aspirin — it can therefore be used as a painkiller. The beauty of this analysis is that it has also shown that Meadowsweet contains tannin and mucilage, both of which act to protect the lining of the stomach. Hence, Meadowsweet does not produce the side effects seen when synthetic aspirin is used. Remedies based on chemicals will never compare with the beauty and intelligence of natural medicines. Daniel Mowrey's excellent book, *The Scientific Validation of Herbal Medicine*, should convince even the most sceptical reader of the validity of herbal medicine.

Table 6.1 below briefly compares conventional and herbal medicine.

Table 6.1 Conventional drugs vs. herbal medicines

Conventional drugs	Herbal medicines
Based on isolated chemicals	Based on the whole plant
Many now made synthetically	All are natural

Not part of the natural energy cycle and so are deficient in energy	All are energy-rich as they use the sun's energy
Use unnaturally high concentrations of a chemical which can disturb a natural system like the body, causing side effects	Use natural concentrations and so are much safer for the body
Are more dramatic in their action as they enter the bloodstream rapidly	Are slower to work
Lower the vitality of the body and increase the work of elimination	Enhance the vitality of the body by providing minerals and vitamins

Herbal Medicine and Intuition

Nature intended us to use herbs to heal ourselves. Everything we need to heal ourselves is provided by Nature. If a dog has eaten meat that has gone off, it will take some couchgrass (*Agropyron repens*) to make itself vomit. It knows instinctively which plant to eat to treat itself. Likewise, primitive people know which plants to use to cure different ailments. Our ancestors had a similar wealth of knowledge which was handed down from generation to generation. This intuitive knowledge must be respected. Science has tried to diminish its importance and to substitute analysis for intuition. We know instinctively what our bodies need to stay healthy. Trusting these instincts is not so easy, however. As children we were not encouraged to be trusting, so we find this very difficult as adults.

Natural medicine is more an art than a science. Doctors, therapists and healers must have a well-developed sense of intuition to work in this area. The reverse is true of conventional medicine which has allowed itself to become very scientific. A marriage of the two can result in a harmony between art and science, between intuitive ability and scientific skills.

Let's take a look at particular herbs which have proven to be successful at treating anxiety and depression and which can aid in the withdrawal from the BZs.

I shall firstly discuss the best anti-anxiety herb (probably even the best natural medicine), kava kava. Because anxiety and depression are often linked, I shall then go on to discuss a powerful natural antidepressant, Hypericum perforatum or St John's Wort, which has not only attracted the attention of the medical profession, because it has been proven to be effective in many clinical trials, but is attracting a lot of media attention, mainly because Prozac and other antidepressants have so many side effects while St John's Wort is virtually side-effect-free. Then I shall discuss herbs which are helpful in easing the withdrawal from the BZs.

Kava Kava (Piper Methysticum)

INTRODUCTION

This must rank as the most magical of all the herbs used to treat the nervous system. Everyone in the Western world should use this herb, either by itself or in combination with other herbs, to help cope with the stress of modern life. This herb acts in a similar way to the BZs, in that it has a strong calming effect, can be used to induce sleep, and is a muscle relaxant. It is different to the BZs in that it calms the mind but also enhances mental activity; it does not have the side effects of the BZs (hangover, dependence, etc.) and does not lose its effectiveness with time. It is also helping medical researchers as most of the laboratory models used to explain how a substance produces a calming effect are simply not sufficient to explain the effects of kava kava. Kava kava also has very unusual, pharmacological properties which I shall explain later. All in all it is a fascinating medicine when one considers that it has a proven calming effect equal to the BZs with none of the side effects of these drugs. Having studied the research on this herb and having used it over the last few years, I can recommend it without hesitation. Let's look at it in more detail now.

GENERAL DESCRIPTION

This herb is indigenous to the South Sea Islands or Oceania. It is an attractive shrub that can attain heights of more than three metres and is a member of the pepper family. It is the root of the plant which is used for medical purposes.

Kava kava is used by the Polynesians as a beverage before meals to help one relax in the same way that we would use alcohol. It is also used to resolve disputes between people and at special social events, e.g. weddings, because of its calming effect and capacity to promote sociability. It also has powerful medicinal usage and is a favourite among the healers of Oceania.

It was introduced to Europe by Captain James Cook after his voyage to the South Seas in 1768. The preparation of the extract of kava kava was described in 1784 by Georg Förster, a young naturalist on Captain Cook's second Pacific voyage. The natives of the South Sea Islands mix the juice from the roots of the plant with coconut milk and then drink it.

PHARMACOLOGY

This herb has been the subject of scientific research for over 100 years. The identification of the first active ingredient was made in 1889. Today it is accepted that a group of chemical compounds known as kavalactones are responsible for the beneficial effects of this plant. All in all, a total of fifteen kavalactones have been isolated and identified and six of these have been chemically synthesised.

Many of the studies on the activity of kavalactones were conducted by a team of scientists from the Freiberg University Institute of Pharmacology in Germany during the 1950s and 1960s. This research has verified that kavalactones do indeed exhibit sedative, muscle relaxant, analgesic and anticonvulsant effects.

More recent studies from the University of New South Wales in Australia have shown that kavalactones exert many of their effects in an unusual way. For example, most sedative drugs, such as the BZs, work by binding to specific receptor sites in the brain, which then leads to chemical changes that promote sedation. Kavalactones do not bind to these same receptors but by some mechanism as yet unexplained they produce almost identical effects. Other studies indicate that kavalactones may act on the limbic system — an ancient part of the brain that affects all other brain activities and is the seat of the emotions. It would appear that kavalactones calm the physical body and the mind and have a stabilising effect on one's emotions. It may be that the primary site of action of kava kava is on the limbic system or one's emotions and from there it exerts a calming effect on the rest of the brain.

Another interesting characteristic of kava kava compared to the BZs is that unlike those drugs it does not lose effectiveness with time and you do not have to take more of it over time to achieve the same effect, which again demonstrates the unusual properties of this herb.

CLINICAL APPLICATION
On the basis of the large amount of research done on kava kava, several European countries have approved its use in the treatment of nervous anxiety, insomnia and restlessness.

One double-blind study (i.e. one in which neither doctor nor patient knows which substance is being used) compared the effect of one of the BZs, oxazepam, to kavain (one of the kavalactones) in the treatment of anxiety. The results showed that 500 mg of kavain daily was as effective as oxazepam. While oxazepam has serious side effects and is addictive, kavain was free of these effects. Another double-blind study came to the same conclusion but also showed that kavain had the ability to improve mental function — in particular it improved memory, reaction time and word recognition. This effect is very interesting as all the conventional BZs decrease mental function, even to the point of making driving and working with dangerous machinery a problem. Very obviously, kava kava is a much safer substance to use as a sedative.

The German Federal Health Agency produced a monograph on kava kava in January 1990 after doing an extensive review of the literature. This monograph approved the use of kava kava as a natural sedative. The main contraindications were pregnancy, breastfeeding and endogenous depression. Kava kava was also shown to be free of any serious side effect. Temporary yellow discoloration of skin/hair/nails was the only mentioned side effect of note, with rare allergic skin rash. It is a very safe herb to use. It is advised not to use kava kava with alcohol, barbiturates or benzodiazepines as the sedative effect may be too strong. The recommended dosage is 60–120 mg of kavalactone, which is equivalent to three to six standard herbal capsules (350 mg pure herb).

The main uses of this herb are as follows:

- for anxiety — it is superior to the BZs in the treatment of anxiety in that it is virtually free of side effects, does not lose effectiveness with time and is not addictive
- for muscle spasm
- for pain relief — superior to aspirin

The studies on kava kava's painkilling ability indicate that it reduces pain in a manner unlike any of the conventional painkillers such as morphine, codeine, the anti-inflammatories (aspirin, brufen, ponstan). This supports the view that modern scientific models to explain how painkillers act to reduce pain in the body are inadequate. This herb is opening the way to more novel research.

A less well-known activity of kava kava is its usefulness in helping the brain tissue recover from the effects of a stroke. Kava kava appears to be able to protect against brain damage due to ischaemia. Kavalactones have been shown to limit the area of damage caused by a stroke; they also have a mild anticonvulsant effect. So if you have had a stroke or are at risk of one, kava kava is well worth taking on a regular basis.

In the South Seas kava kava is referred to as the plant of 'knowledge', i.e. it helps one to know oneself. Because it produces deep relaxation on a physical level and a calm but heightened state of mental awareness, it can give one greater access to the deeper, emotional and spiritual aspects of oneself. The indigenous healers of the South Pacific use this herb to access their higher or spiritual selves. Fijian healers use it to gain insights into which medicines to use to help their patients. It is also taken at night to gain access to the dream state, as kava kava will produce more vivid, lucid dreams.

This is a herb that is of immense value for its medicinal benefits but also for gaining insights into the deeper aspects of our being.

Hypericum Perforatum (St John's Wort)

INTRODUCTION

This is a plant that doesn't need introducing to Europeans as it grows freely throughout the grasslands and woodlands of much of Western Europe. The plant owes its name to the fact that it flowers around the time of 'St John's Tide' or the summer solstice, producing beautiful yellow flowers.

Hypericum is mentioned in many ancient medical texts. It has become famous for its mood-enhancing abilities as well as its antiviral effects, to the point where conventional medicine can no longer ignore it. It is now playing an important role by bridging the gap between conventional and alternative medicine. This is due to the fact that numerous clinical trials have demonstrated its effectiveness and many doctors in Europe are now prescribing it.

It has become extremely popular in Western Europe over the last fifteen years as a natural antidepressant. In Germany doctors write over three million prescriptions per year, which represents twenty-five times the number they write for Prozac. Clearly this herb is gaining the upper hand over its synthetic rival. Its popularity is gaining rapidly in North America, where it is now being described as the ideal treatment for mild to moderate depression as it has proven efficacy and proven safety. It also has anti-anxiety, or sedative, properties. All the major manufacturers of natural medicine are now investing in and marketing hypericum.

How It Works

The active constituents found in hypericum are a group of compounds called hypericins — one is called hypericin, another pseudohypericin and another hyperforim.

The hypericins were initially thought to work as monoamine oxidose inhibitors[1] (MAOIs) but this model is inadequate in terms of explaining the mode of action of hypericum. There are other active constituents in the herb which do not work as MAOIs, which makes it all the more important to use the whole herb and not the isolated hypericins alone. Actually, this truth applies to most herbal substances.

What Is It Used For?

1. Depression

Most research to date has centred on its usage as an antidepressant. It seems to be most effective for mild/moderate depression but not so useful for endogenous depression, nor for manic depression.

The *Journal of Geriatric Psychiatry and Neurology* in 1994 devoted seventeen research papers to hypericum. One particular story tracked 3,250 patients with mild to moderate depression and showed an 80 per cent improvement after a mere four weeks of treatment.

[1] Antidepressants work by increasing the level of certain chemicals in the brain, e.g. serotonin, noradrenalin or dopamine, either by preventing their re-uptake into the nerve endings or by inhibiting their breakdown by certain enzymes, one of which is monoamine oxidose.

Dr David Linde et al. reviewed twenty-three clinical trials involving 1,757 patients and the results demonstrated that hypericum was three times more effective than the placebo. These results were reported in the *British Medical Journal* in August 1996. Other trials have shown that the antidepressant effects of hypericum were comparable or superior to standard pharmaceutical drugs such as imipramine.

There are many other trials demonstrating the efficiency of this herb, to the point where the National Institutes for Health and the National Institutes for Mental Health in the USA are planning a large multi-centre trial of this herb in the treatment of mild/moderate depression. The NIH and the NIMH are both government bodies and have at last acknowledged the importance of herbs in the treatment of medical conditions.

2. ANTIVIRAL

Hypericum has long been known to have anti-infective properties but it is only more recently that scientific studies have validated this claim. In a series of nine studies, extracts of hypericum were tested against streptococcal infections and found to be more effective than the sulpha antibiotics, e.g. bactrim, septrin.

There is now significant interest in its antiviral activity. Research to date indicates that there is a degree of direct antiviral action. As a result of this it is being tested in HIV and Hepatitis C infections.

3. SEDATIVE

Hypericum does not appear to have strong sedative properties, yet many textbooks on herbal medicine state that it does have mild to moderate sedative effects. Most of the research done centres on its antidepressant or mood-elevating effects. I think it is best therefore to regard this herb as an important natural antidepressant, rather than as a sedative.

IS IT SAFE?

It is a safe herb. There have been no reported deaths.

Approximately 2 per cent of patients in the above-mentioned clinical trials reported side effects, mainly in the form of mild gastro-intestinal irritation. This makes it the treatment of choice in mild to moderate depression. When one compares it to the conventional antidepressants such as Prozac, which has significant side effects (insomnia, loss of weight, sexual dysfunction), it is no wonder that many doctors are now turning to hypericum to treat depression.

On searching the literature for other side effects associated with the use of St John's Wort, two points are worthy of mention. Firstly, there is the potential for a photosensitivity reaction following *external* application in humans. This reaction can take the form of hives through to dermatitis following exposure of the area to sunlight, after applying Hypericum perforatum to the skin. When it is used internally in humans, photosensitivity reactions are very rare, especially if the herb is used at normal therapeutic doses. The photosensitive reaction St John's Wort provokes in livestock is considered to be a problem of economic importance, particularly in Australia, where cattle and sheep may ingest large quantities of the herb and as a consequence develop swelling of the ears, eyes and face from scratching these areas.

Secondly, internal use of Hypericum perforatum may alter milk production in lactating mothers. The flavour of the milk may be changed and the milk may be reduced in quantity or may cease altogether.

DOSAGE RANGES OF HYPERICUM PERFORATUM
(from the *British Herbal Pharmacopoeia*)
If using St John's Wort as a liquid extract, use two to four millilitres three times daily. If using the whole herb in dried form, use two to four grams daily.

Standard dried extract is a common form in which to find it in health food shops. Use approximately 350 mg two to three times daily but do not exceed 1,000 mg daily.

It takes anything up to two to three weeks to feel the benefit of the herb so be patient; at least you don't have to endure the side effects associated with conventional antidepressants.

Herbs which Assist with the Withdrawal from the BZs

When discussing herbs which relax the nervous system, I have to mention two in particular. One of these is skullcap (Scutellaria laterifolia). Its main action is as a sedative and it probably ranks as the most widely used nerve relaxant worldwide. It is famous for its ability to relax states of nervous tension while renewing and reviving nervous tissue at the same time. I personally have used it very successfully in the treatment of tension headaches and anxiety.

Because of its calming and nourishing effect on the central nervous system, it has a powerful role to play in assisting patients to withdraw from the BZs. In this role it is often combined with a second herb, Valerian. This herb has been recognised as a sedative in conventional medical pharmacopoeias and many of the older pharmacists know of its ability to treat nervous disorders. However, Valerian has certain disadvantages in that (a) it does not suit everyone, (b) it has a very strong odour, (c) it is suggested by some that it may become habit-forming and (d) if taken continuously for a long period of time, e.g. more than six months, it can cause nerve damage.

Because of Valerian's therapeutic value it is often combined with skullcap to help strengthen the nervous system for a three-month period and is then replaced with other herbs such as hops, catnip, lavender or ginseng.

How to Use Skullcap and Valerian

If you suffer from nervous tension or are trying to withdraw from one of the BZs, use a mixture of skullcap and valerian for a period of three months. Use a tincture (liquid extract) of both herbs and mix them in equal parts. Shake the mixture well each time you use it. Use anything from ten to fifteen drops of this mixture three times daily in a little water. It is best taken on an empty stomach.

Most people are able to withdraw from a tranquilliser within three months. However, after withdrawal it may take another six to twelve months for the nervous system to recover completely so continue to use herbal tonics to assist during this period. There are many good nerve tonics on the market but one of the best I've seen is a substance called Nervol. It contains skullcap in combination with oat, vervain and catnip. Oat is good for nourishing the nervous system, especially in times of stress, and vervain tones and strengthens the whole nervous system while having a mild sedative effect. Catnip (Nepeta cataria) was prized in Roman times for its medicinal properties. The dried leaves were smoked as a way of relieving the pressures of life. Today its sedative properties are well recognised.

Nervol can be used in states of nervous tension and after a valerian/skullcap combination in the withdrawal from central nervous system drugs such as the BZs and antidepressants. In tablet form it is best used as one tablet, three times daily, or in tincture form as ten to fifteen drops, three times daily in a little water. The herbs used in the production of Nervol are grown organically and the extract is then energised in a special way so as to boost its therapeutic effect. It is a rather unique product and one well worth using if under stress or if withdrawing from any nervous system drug, e.g. tranquillisers, sleeping pills or antidepressants.

Summary

Kava kava is one of the most important herbs of our times. It is gaining a wonderful reputation for its calming and tension-relieving properties. However, it has many added benefits as a muscle relaxant, painkiller and protector against cerebral ischaemia (stroke).

This herb is attracting a lot of interest from the scientific and medical community as its mode of action has scientists amazed. It does not conform to any of the models that scientists use to explain how either (a) sedative substances or (b) painkillers work on the central nervous system. It is a beautiful example of how Nature is challenging our limited medical models of how the body works.

Because kava kava has such a powerful relaxant effect on the physical and mental bodies, much like hypnosis, it can allow one to see the cause of one's anxiety difficulties, which often reside in the emotional or spiritual bodies. Kava kava also enhances the dream state, so giving greater insights into one's life.

This is a truly remarkable herb, with none of the side effects associated with the BZs and other central nervous system drugs.

Hypericum perforatum is another herb that is attracting a great deal of interest across the Western world as it has proven to be as effective as some of the pharmaceutical antidepressants without the serious side effects. Countless studies have been carried out in both England and Germany which have convinced many doctors, to the point where it is fast becoming the main form of treatment for mild to moderate depression. This herb is truly bridging the gap between two forms of medicine — the old and the new, between the natural world and modern scientific research. It also has proven antiviral effects.

The future for this herb is promising as the National Institutes for Health and the National Institutes for Mental Health are planning a large trial to assess its role in the treatment of depression in the USA. It is an extremely safe herb to use, especially in therapeutic doses.

When withdrawing from a benzodiazepine tranquilliser use skullcap and valerian for three months and then use skullcap in combination with other nerve tonics such as oat, catnip and vervain, as in the product Nervol, for another six to twelve months at least.

7   Homoeopathy

Introduction

The way the body can heal itself is miraculous. When you cut yourself accidentally you don't have to think about how the wound is going to heal; the body's own inner healer gets to work and within a few days the wound is well healed. Every day the body staves off innumerable infective agents and adapts to many stresses. This inner intelligence works continuously without you being aware of it.

Conventional doctors know about this inner wisdom but choose to ignore it for the most part. There is a belief among medical scientists and doctors that they know more and so they force the body to heal in a particular way; homoeopathy rather assists the body's own inner healing powers. The main flaw in conventional medical thinking is that doctors tend to assume that the symptoms represent the disease and when these symptoms are controlled, eliminated or suppressed, the disease will disappear. For example, if you have a fever and a cough, paracetamol is used to control the fever while a codeine-based cough remedy will suppress the cough reflex.

Every other form of medicine views symptoms in a different light. The word 'symptom' is derived from Greek and means 'signal' or 'sign'. Symptoms are signals or signs of the body's own inner healer at work, e.g. the body will raise its temperature in response to an infection to prevent an invading bacterium from surviving — most bacteria cannot survive at higher temperatures. Similarly a cough is the body trying to expel an irritant, e.g. virus, dust, smoke, allergen; suppressing the cough ensures that the irritant will remain in the body and cause further damage. Homoeopathy is a system of medicine which stimulates the body's own healing powers; it stimulates symptoms and so helps the body's inner healer.

The Basis of Homoeopathy

1. PRINCIPLE OF SIMILARS

Homoeopathic medicine is based on the principle of similars — that is, whatever symptoms a remedy causes in large doses, it can heal when given in extremely small doses. Conventional medicine also applies this principle of similars in two instances: (a) desensitising a patient to an allergen and (b) immunising against an infection. Giving small doses of bacteria or viruses has been found to stimulate a person's immunity against these bacteria or viruses and giving small doses of an allergen helps the body's defences to cope with large amounts of a particular allergen. In homoeopathy, belladonna and aconitum are two substances that cause fever when given in large doses and help to resolve a fever when given in very small doses — the principle of similars!

2. SMALL DOSES

Homoeopathic medicines are specially prepared small doses of mainly plant (e.g. belladonna) and mineral (e.g. sulphur) substances which undergo a specific process of dilution with water (with or without alcohol) and succussion (vigorous shaking). A substance is diluted one part to nine parts water (1:10 dilution) or one part to ninety-nine parts water (1:100 dilution) and shaken (succussed), then diluted again and shaken and the process is repeated.

A 1:10 dilution is given the symbol 'x' and a 1:100 dilution the symbol 'C' (from the Roman numerals for these numbers). If a substance is diluted 1:10 six times it is given the symbol 6x. This process of successive dilution and succussion is called potentisation. Hence you will recognise homoeopathic medicines as the potency (e.g. 6x) will be written after the name of the substance, e.g. Belladonna 6x or Sulphur 6c.

Interestingly, the more a substance is diluted and succussed the more *potent* it becomes. Many conventionally trained pharmacists and doctors have great difficulty believing this statement and in truth it has been the source of fascination among practitioners and researchers in the field of homoeopathy, especially if one considers that highly diluted homoeopathic remedies may contain no trace of the original substance. In fact, a homoeopathic remedy over the 24x potency (twenty-four successive dilutions and succussions) will have no molecules of the original substance remaining. These higher potencies are merely water or a mixture of water and alcohol. So how can these potencies work?

According to Dr Trevor Cook, President of the United Kingdom Homoeopathic Medical Association, the explanation appears to lie in the field of quantum physics. It is known that all matter consists of and radiates energy. Some substances, such as plutonium, radiate a great deal of energy; each substance radiates this energy at a particular frequency. Some frequencies are harmful to the body, e.g. plutonium, while others are helpful.

In the same way that a cassette tape can store the notes (frequencies) of a song, scientists have discovered that water can store the frequency of a substance with which it is mixed. The more the substance is succussed or shaken, the more water molecules store the frequency, i.e. the water molecules begin to radiate the frequency of the original substance. In other words, water begins to mimic the original substance with which it is mixed and begins to behave as if it were that substance. The more water molecules that do this, the more potent the effect. This would explain how higher potencies have a stronger therapeutic effect even though they have little or none of the original substance in them.

A lot of sceptics assert that homoeopathic medicines have such low doses of a therapeutic substance that they cannot work. These people are usually unaware of the wide body of clinical studies and clinical experience which clearly validates the case that homoeopathy is an effective form of medicine. There is a huge volume of medical literature supporting homoeopathy but I shall mention just a few articles to illustrate the point that homoeopathy works.

In 1991 three professors of medicine analysed twenty-five years of clinical studies using homoeopathic medicines and published their results (J. Kleijnen et al., *British Medical Journal,* February 1991, 302: 316–23). This analysis covered 107 trials and over 80 per cent of these showed that homoeopathy was effective. The studies varied a lot in the way they were designed but the professors concluded that the better designed and performed the studies were, the higher the likelihood that the medicines were found to be effective. They admitted that 'the amount of positive results came as a surprise to us'. The studies showed that homoeopathy was beneficial in treating headaches, respiratory infections, digestive disorders, hay fever, arthritis and psychological problems, along with a host of other complaints.

A double-blind study involving 478 patients suffering from flu was conducted in the UK in 1989 (P. Farley et al., *British Journal of Clinical Pharmacology,* March 1989, 27: 329–35). This study was looking at the effectiveness of a well-known French homoeopathic remedy known as Oscillococcinum. The trial showed that almost twice as many people who took the homoeopathic remedy got over the flu after forty-eight hours as compared to those given a placebo. This remedy was more effective in people under the age of thirty than for those over thirty.

Homoeopathy vs. Tranquillisers

One of the reasons why homoeopaths commonly experience good results in treating emotional ailments is because homoeopathy is an integrated system which can heal the emotional, mental and physical aspects of an illness concurrently. To quote George Vithoulkas, a well-known author and teacher of homoeopathy:

'The long-term benefit of homoeopathy is that it not only alleviates the presenting symptoms but it re-establishes internal order at the deepest levels and thereby provides a lasting cure.' The secret in treating patients' complaints using homoeopathy is to get the right remedy in the right potency, when using single remedies, or to choose the appropriate complex remedy when using complex homoeopathy.

A simple remedy is one substance prepared as a single potency, e.g. Belladonna 6x. If we then mix Belladonna 6x with Belladonna 30x, this becomes a complex remedy; similarly, if we mix Belladonna 6x with Echinacea 6x, it becomes a complex remedy. So, a complex remedy is a *mixture* of either the same substance in different potencies or different substances, regardless of the potencies.

I shall discuss first some simple remedies which are often used to treat emotional disturbances, and later deal with some complex remedies.

Homoeopathic Remedies and Nervous Disorders

1. SINGLE HOMOEOPATHIC REMEDIES
The main reason for prescribing tranquillisers such as the benzodiazepines (BZs) is for the relief of either acute or chronic anxiety. There are many good single homoeopathic remedies which can help in such situations.

Gelsemium. If anxiety causes a paralysing feeling in you, where you can't move or think, with tremors or headache, then this may be the remedy for you. It is often used to help people with stage fright or before an exam or a sports event. It is also used for the effects of bad news or grief, for deep-seated fears and for where excitement causes diarrhoea.

There are varying opinions on how to choose the best potency. A simple rule of thumb is that if you are uncertain about the suitability of the remedy use a lower potency, e.g. 6x or 12x (or 6c or 12c), and if you are more certain use the 30x or 30c potency.

Other general guidelines are as follows:

- If the onset of symptoms is rapid use a higher potency, 30x or 30c.
- If a person is very allergic use a lower potency.
- The cardinal rule is 'minimum dosage', i.e. once the person shows improvement, decrease the dose or frequency of dosage and stop shortly afterwards. Taking homoeopathic remedies long-term is unnecessary.

Argentum Nitricum. This substance is useful for severe anxiety or nervous tension, especially if there is profound anticipation about what might happen. It is described in many homoeopathic texts as one of the great remedies for the terror of anticipation. Patients for whom the remedy is suitable may also experience claustrophobia. They also have fears of being alone or of death. They often deal with their anxiety by walking faster and faster and so exhaust themselves.

Again use a 6 potency (i.e. 6x or 6c) if you are unsure, a 12 potency if you are more certain and a 30 or higher potency if you are very sure. Potencies greater than a 30x or 30c are not available over the counter and need a homoeopathic prescription.

Lycopodium. This remedy is helpful for people with lots of fears — fear of crowds, of the dark, of death, of ghosts, of people. These people tend to wake up in bad mood. They are often intellectuals who have low self-esteem, and are particularly afraid of appearing foolish or incompetent.

Case History — James: Age Thirty Years

James was marketing manager of a medium-sized company in Dublin. He was outwardly very confident, polite and accommodating. He came to me complaining of upper abdominal discomfort especially after eating a meal, when he got a lot of bloating and wind. He found that his symptoms were worse before having to attend a meeting, especially when he had to speak in front of others. Often he couldn't eat for some time after such meetings as he got quite worked up or anxious. His symptoms were noticeably worse in the afternoons.

I treated him with Lycopodium 30c initially to see how he would respond. Three weeks later on his second visit he reported that his symptoms had improved but not gone. I then used Lycopodium 200c and the response was quite dramatic. His physical symptoms disappeared and he reported less anxiety associated with public speaking.

Lycopodium patients are often outwardly quite confident but inwardly feel weak and inadequate.

Characteristic symptoms which often reveal the need for lycopodium are where the patient's symptoms are worse in the afternoon between four and eight, craving sweets, lots of dyspepsia and wind, and abdominal bloating. If you identify with these symptoms, then use lycopodium in a 6x or 30x potency depending upon your level of certainty.

Dosage: The following dosage applies to each of the above-mentioned single remedies. If using tablets the dosage is one tablet for an adult and if using drops the dosage is ten drops for anyone over the age of sixteen. For anyone between the ages of six and sixteen, use half the adult dose, and for younger children consult a homoeopathic practitioner or homoeopathic pharmacist.

2. COMPLEX HOMOEOPATHIC REMEDIES

Ignatia Homaccord. This is particularly useful where there is acute anxiety or grief as in the death of a loved one, break-up in a close relationship, sudden shock or disappointment. Where there is a tendency to weep, frequent sighs, a lump in the throat and headache, this remedy is especially suitable.

This complex remedy contains two main substances in both low and high potencies. One of these is Ignatia, which is best used for acute conditions. (If the condition recurs again and again Natrum muriaticum is a better remedy.) The other constituent of this medicine is Moschus, which is suitable for conditions of nervous excitability, restlessness, and acute anxiety associated with palpitations. All in all, this is an excellent remedy for situations that arise in all our lives that are difficult to handle emotionally. This substance comes in the form of drops and injection solution.

Dosage: If using the drops take ten drops six times daily for the first day and then ten drops three times daily; however, if the anxiety is particularly acute take ten drops every half-hour until an improvement is noticed and then use ten drops three times daily, or it may be better to use this remedy in injection form. In either case it is wiser to consult a practitioner or pharmacist who is qualified to advise you about homoeopathic medicines.

Case History — Mary: Age Twenty-Five Years

Mary had a five-year relationship with her boyfriend Paul, with whom she was living. She described their relationship as very close and she believed that they were destined to spend the rest of their lives together. When they broke up she came to see me complaining of severe tightness in the chest, causing her difficulty in breathing. She explained that the symptoms began with the break-up in her relationship with her boyfriend; at this point she began crying and she spent most of the consultation weeping.

I prescribed Ignatia 30c and asked her to come and see me in one week. On her return she was still emotionally fragile but her physical symptoms were gone completely and she was able to breathe normally.

It is sometimes hard to distinguish between the two homoeopathic remedies Ignatia and Natrum muriaticum. In many ways the two remedies are identical. In general, Nat. mur. patients can tolerate more emotional stress without breaking down; patients for whom Ignatia is the better remedy are emotionally weaker and can break down with relatively minor stresses. As a consequence, Ignatia patients cry more easily and often sigh a lot. Personally, this is my way of being able to distinguish between the two remedies.

Neuro Injeel. This is another complex remedy commonly used for a range of mental or emotional conditions. This remedy contains the following constituents:

- Acidum phosphorium — for physical and mental exhaustion
- Argentum nitricum — for anxiety, fears and melancholia
- Sepia — for nervous exhaustion, depression, irritability
- Valerian — for anxiety and insomnia
- Avena sativa — for anxiety and insomnia

This remedy also contains Ignatia and so is a more broad-spectrum treatment than Ignatia Homaccord. Because of the sepia and Acidum phosphoricum, it is particularly useful when the patient has reached a point of *exhaustion*. It is also of use where one is trying to withdraw from nicotine, alcohol or tranquillisers. I have used it with great success in treating patients who are withdrawing from the BZs and who get rebound insomnia or rebound anxiety.

Dosage: Because this remedy is available in injection form only, it must be administered by a homoeopathic practitioner.

Summary
Homoeopathy is an integrated system of medicine that can deal with the emotional as well as the physical aspects of an illness concurrently. It aims at restoring an inner harmony in the body so providing a cure for the complaint. In contrast, many of the conventional drugs aim at suppressing symptoms, which homoeopaths regard as the body's own healing power at work.

Classically trained homoeopaths use single remedies, which means one substance in one potency; those trained in complex homoeopathy use complex remedies, which often have a number of constituents in varying potencies. For acute anxiety three simple remedies which can help are gelsemium, argentum nitricum and lycopodium. Two complex remedies of note are

Ignatia Homaccord and Neuro Injeel. The latter is particularly useful when trying to withdraw from tranquillisers; however, it is available only in injection solution.

8 Nutritional Medicine

Eating and breathing are the two most important things we do every day in order to stay alive. The food with which you nourish your body is of critical importance to your health. Good food — natural foods which Nature intended you to eat — will provide your body with the nutrients essential for good health, particularly an effective immune system. Bad food — unnatural or processed foods — will lead to a steady decline in your health, making you more prone to infections.

After almost twelve years in Africa, I was shocked on my return to Europe to see the kind of foods people were eating here. In Africa, people eat a diet based on natural foods, at least for the most part. They eat a minimum of processed foods as they are too expensive. What grows in the back garden is cheap, but what comes from food processing factories is expensive. In Europe, much of the food that we consume is 'dead' food. It contains too much sugar and much of it is processed.

Figure 8.1

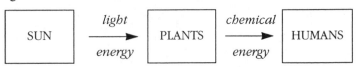

All energy on this planet comes from the sun. The sun provides us with heat and light energy. As Figure 8.1 above shows, plants use light energy from the sun to make food in a process called photosynthesis. During photosynthesis, light energy is converted to chemical energy. This energy is passed along to us when we eat the plant. Hence, we refer to natural foods as being energy-rich. Put simply, the sun's energy ends up in your body, keeping it healthy.

Humans are part of an energy pathway which can be demonstrated in the following diagram.

Figure 8.2

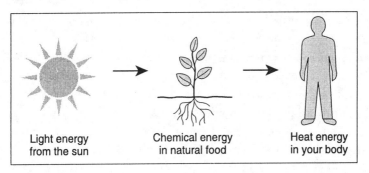

Light energy from the sun → Chemical energy in natural food → Heat energy in your body

No small wonder then that so many cultures have worshipped the sun, as it is truly the giver of life on this planet.

Much of the food we eat, however, is removed from this energy pathway and processed in a factory. Unnatural chemicals are often added, such as flavourings, colourings or preservatives. The food is depleted of its natural energy, it is 'dead' so to speak. It is also toxic for the body due to the presence of these additives and this increases the work of elimination from the body.

The message is simple — the closer your food is to Nature, the higher its energy content and the healthier your body will be.

Water
Water is the body's single most important nutrient. Approximately 60 per cent of the human body consists of water, so we should remember to drink lots of it daily. It is

recommended that a 50 kg woman should drink approximately 1–2 litres daily. A 70 kg man should consume 2–3 litres per day.

While these quantities are just guidelines, the most important thing is to listen to your own body. When you are thirsty, drink water — but make sure it's safe water! Filtered or fresh spring water is best, although bottled is better than tap water.

The quality of our water supplies has become a major public health issue. Children seem to know instinctively that tap water is unsuitable for drinking — the odour and taste probably give them instant clues. Many children in modern cities and towns take in the bulk of their fluid requirements from soft drinks rather than water. Soft drinks are composed of carbonated water to which flavourings, colourings and other substances are added. In many cities, tap water is not only foul-tasting and foul-smelling, it also contains chlorine, fluoride, heavy metals and other chemicals which are potentially harmful to the body. If your pets are not willing to drink it, treat it with suspicion.

Chlorine is used to kill harmful bacteria in the water supply (this is why it's added to swimming pools). But chlorine will also kill some of the 'good' bacteria in the human digestive system. Chlorine has been found to provoke asthmatic attacks and to contribute to arteriosclerosis (hardening of the arteries).

Fluoride is another substance commonly added to the water supply in many countries. While it is intended to prevent tooth decay, fluoride has been shown to damage brain and nerve cells and to cause liver damage. It creates a high incidence of bone fractures as well. Fluoride stimulates bone formation but the bone is often poorly mineralised and therefore more liable to fracture.

When I was a child in Northern Ireland, we lived in the countryside and had a well in our back garden. This was our main source of water for a number of years. Since few chemical insecticides and pesticides were used on the soil in those days, the water was pure and safe to drink. It came straight from Nature. Now, however, reports of the chemical analyses done on the water table in different parts of Europe leave one in no doubt about the damage done to our precious water supplies over the last forty years. As a result, we are forced to consume either filtered water or bottled water.

In the late 1960s, we went on a school trip to France. I was surprised to see so many people drinking water from a bottle, as I had never seen bottled water before. Today, bottled water is commonplace the world over. This is a reflection of how unsafe our water supplies have become.

In Africa, water is a life-and-death issue. Due to the contamination of the water supply, a significant percentage of children do not make it through their first year of life — many die from gastroenteritis and other water-borne diseases. A safe water supply is the key to the health of a whole village or community in Africa. Unfortunately, the same is becoming true in Europe. The most basic of all nutrients, water, is now becoming unsafe to drink.

Refined Carbohydrates

The amount of sugar consumed by the average adult and child in the Western world is indeed worrying. When shopping in the supermarkets of Europe, it is alarming to see just how many of the foods contain sugar. Most breakfast cereals contain sugar — a bowl of muesli may contain the equivalent of two tablespoons of sugar. Soft drinks also have a high sugar content — Lucozade and Coca-Cola contain the equivalent of seven teaspoons of sugar per glass (200 ml)! These examples show how important it is to read the labels on all processed foods. If you wish to know the quantity of any of the constituents of a particular food item, write to the manufacturer.

Refined sugar, like refined flour, is a product of Western civilisation. It's an *unnatural* food and, so, completely unnecessary in the diet. Worse still, it contributes to ill health. Over 150 years ago, Native American Indians warned of the harmful effects of refined sugar on the body. They observed that the white man ate too many sweet things, which weakened the body. Today, those words are proving to be all too true.

Sugar encourages the growth of a number of bacteria and fungi

— it is a wonderful growth medium for these micro-organisms. As a result, a diet rich in sweet things may predispose a person to infections. Sugar consumption is associated with tooth decay, candidiasis and mucus production, especially in people predisposed to respiratory problems, such as asthmatics. Many people are now addicted to sugar. As with cigarettes, it can become very difficult to live without it.

In one study by Sanchez et al. in 1973 ('Role of sugar in human neutrophilic phagocytosis', *American Journal of Clinical Nutrition*, 26:180), a high intake of sugar was found to have a negative effect on the immune system. These researchers showed that sugar impaired the ability of white blood cells to gobble up and kill bacteria. This research followed the work of an American physician, Dr B. P. Sandler, who, while working with victims of the polio epidemic in the late 1940s, became convinced that a high sugar intake made one more susceptible to this disease. The 1973 research supported Dr Sandler's hypothesis, as refined sugar was clearly found to suppress the immune system. Other studies have shown that sugar robs the body of certain nutrients, including zinc, which is vital for immune function.

The best sugar is always that which is found in Nature, especially in fresh or dried fruits. Raisins, sultanas and dates are excellent sources of sugar and can be used instead of sugar to sweeten breakfast cereal. Many Africans chew on raw cane sugar and do not suffer the health problems that we do in the West. This may be because eating the natural substance supplies the body with minerals such as calcium, whereas eating refined sugar can rob the body of calcium.

Sugar has a detrimental effect on the health of all of us, but most especially on young children who often consume excessive amounts. Many of the children attending my clinic suffer from recurrent infections, asthma and eczema. An alarming number of them are also deficient in various minerals. The first thing I recommend for these children is a reduction in sugar intake. Some are in such a poor state of health that it is necessary to cut out all sugars for a limited period, thereby allowing their young bodies to recover. The benefits of this treatment are almost immediate. There is an increase in both appetite and energy levels. The whole body starts to function better.

Among the adults that I see, there is almost an epidemic of fungal infections, skin rashes and intestinal candidiasis. Many of these infections improve when sugar and foods that contain sugar are excluded from the diet.

At public talks I am often asked 'Doesn't the body need sugar?' The answer is 'Yes, it does' — but not in the form of unnatural sugars such as glucose, dextrose and sucrose, taken in large quantities on a regular basis. The sugar in fruit and honey — fructose — is natural and much healthier. And remember, starchy foods such as potatoes and rice consist of long chains of glucose molecules. These chains are slowly broken down by the digestive system and glucose is gradually absorbed into the bloodstream.

Figure 8.3 Effects of starch and refined sugar on the body

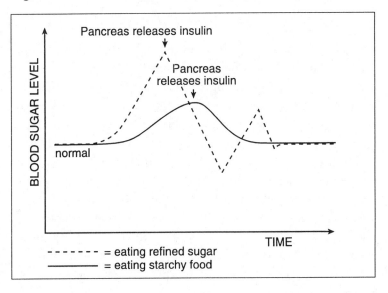

Look at the two graphs in Figure 8.3. When natural foods containing starch are eaten, the blood sugar level rises gradually

(solid line). When this reaches a certain point the pancreas releases insulin and the blood sugar level slowly drops back to normal. In contrast to this, eating foods rich in refined sugar (such as sweets) causes high levels of glucose to enter the bloodstream rapidly (dashed line). This puts stress on the pancreas and it is forced to release large quantities of insulin, as too much sugar in the bloodstream can be dangerous (hyperglycaemia).

The ups and downs in the blood sugar level which occur when sugary foods are consumed disturb the body. They put stress on the pancreas and adrenal glands (secrete adrenaline) and can cause the blood sugar level to drop below normal (hypoglycaemia), as shown by the troughs in the graph. Eating sugary foods occasionally does not cause too much difficulty — it is only when the pancreas and adrenal glands are constantly stressed that problems arise. Avoid such difficulties by eating only natural foods and avoiding sugars that have been bleached, chemically refined and rendered harmful to the body.

Processed Foods
Nature did not intend us to eat from bottles, tins, jars and packets. The body likes food it can digest and assimilate easily. It likes not only protein, carbohydrate and fat in this form, but also vitamins and minerals. Putting natural foods into a natural system makes sense. Ingesting unnatural chemicals, such as those found in processed foods, does not make sense.

During the 1950s and 1960s, processed foods became part of that dubious package sold to people in the West called 'progress'. The country market was replaced by the supermarket in the belief that bigger was better. Even the supermarkets grew up to become hypermarkets. Remember that the primary aim of the food processing industry is profit, not health! It is encouraging to see that country markets are springing up again and that the availability of organically grown foods is on the increase. This trend must be encouraged for the sake of ourselves and our children. Put pressure on your local shop/greengrocer to supply organically grown foods.

The quality of commercially produced cereals, fruits and vegetables has declined considerably in the last ten years. A carrot grown in a market garden near a large city is generally of a much poorer quality than a carrot grown in an unspoilt area. Because of economic pressures, chemicals are used in commercial farming and this results in the depletion of the soil itself. A depleted soil produces depleted, poorer-quality vegetables. All the nutrients that a carrot needs must come from the soil. If the goodness of the soil becomes depleted, because too many crops have been grown too quickly, the soil will lack essential minerals and vitamins. When you eat food grown under these circumstances, your body also becomes deprived of certain nutrients, and so the cycle of mineral/vitamin deficiency begins.

The best-quality cereals, fruits and vegetables come from organic farms, that is farms which do not use chemical fertilisers, chemical pesticides or chemical herbicides and which allow time for the soil to replenish itself between crop cycles.

You can now begin to see why it is important to know how and where your fruits and vegetables are grown. If in doubt, grow your own or buy organically grown produce.

Food Additives
One of the greatest health problems facing the modern world today is the ongoing contamination of our food supply. Governments across the Western world choose to ignore it when the food industry adds very questionable chemicals such as dyes, flavourings, stabilisers and preservatives to our foods, let alone the spraying of foods with pesticides as well as the antibiotics, hormones and other drugs given to commercial animals.

There are over 2,000 food additives licensed for use in the food industry in the EU. Here are some of them with some of the problems that they cause — I shall focus mainly on the central nervous system side effects.

1. YELLOW DYE NO. 5
This is a dye found in sweets, soft drinks, ice cream and pasta. It

can cause life-threatening asthmatic symptoms in certain sensitive people.

2. Yellow Dye No. 6
Used in sweets and soft drinks, this additive has been shown to increase the risk of kidney and adrenal gland tumours in rats. It is also thought to cause chromosomal damage. Because of this evidence, it has been banned in Norway and Sweden.

3. Aspartame (Sold under Trade Names such as Equal, Nutra-Sweet and Canderel)
This is an artificial sweetener to which a number of people are sensitive. Symptoms associated with aspartame sensitivity include depression, headache, nausea, vertigo, insomnia, memory loss and epileptic fits. One should be very careful using such a substance over a long period of time.

4. Saccharin
This is a widely used artificial sweetener and is a possible human carcinogen. It is used in many soft drinks.

5. Nitrites
Nitrites are used as preservatives in cured meats such as bacon, ham and smoked fish. Nitrites are now known to form nitrosomines, which are cancer-causing chemicals, in the gastro-intestinal tract. These chemicals have been associated with human cancer and with birth defects.

6. MSG (Monosodium Glutamate)
This is a flavour enhancer added to most processed foods, takeaway foods and crisps. MSG can alter the chemistry of the brain sufficiently to cause severe headaches, and is one of the main causes of migraine.

I have mentioned only a few of the more commonly used additives with which you may be familiar for the sake of giving you some insight into what you are actually consuming. When you investigate this subject in greater depth you will be left in no doubt about the dangers of a Western diet.

Additives seem to affect so many people, especially children, causing headaches, hyperactivity, irritability and nausea. Many people are unaware of the dangers of food additives, believing that processed and junk foods are safe. The truth is that the quantity added to an individual food item may be safe but when a lot of one particular food additive is consumed or if a number of additives are combined, these chemicals can be toxic. This is why some countries have banned the use of certain food additives — refer to the section on Yellow Dye No. 6 above. It is important that you educate yourself and your family about food additives; a very good book to read is *Additives: A Guide for Everyone* by Eric Milestone and John Abraham (London, Penguin Books: 1988).

Food and Behaviour

Food additives can have a significant effect on behaviour as you can see from some of the above-mentioned examples. There are numerous studies showing that removing food additives and sugar from the diet of prison inmates, or juveniles in reform centres, can curb antisocial behaviour. Similar studies done with schoolchildren have shown an improvement in academic performance when processed and refined foods are removed from the diet.

In much of the literature associated with how food relates to mood, there is a general consensus that refined carbohydrates, especially white sugar (sucrose), can cause depression, irritability and anxiety. This has been more than evident to me over the last ten years of clinical experience. Refined foods deplete the body of B vitamins — the very vitamins the body needs to assimilate sugar. Since vitamin B complex is so essential for the nervous system, it is easy to see why refined carbohydrates can cause nervous disorders such as depression. In addition, refined sugars can stress the pancreas to pump out large amounts of insulin, which will lower blood sugar levels so rapidly that it will cause hypoglycaemia (low blood sugar) attacks. Some of the symptoms associated with low blood sugar include irritability, anxiety and depression.

In addition to robbing the body of B vitamins and stressing the pancreas, refined carbohydrates can cause mood disturbances by altering serotonin levels in the brain.

Your mood depends on the level of certain chemicals in the brain; one of these chemicals is serotonin. When your serotonin level is low your mood is low, and when it is normal your mood is also normal, so one's mood can be directly related to the level of serotonin in the brain. Eating refined carbohydrates causes a temporary rise in the serotonin level, so elevating one's mood. However, this improvement in mood is short-lived, and as soon as the level of serotonin drops, one's mood drops with it. One is often tempted then to consume more refined carbohydrates to get a 'high' again. This is how one can so easily get addicted to sugary foods — one craves them to improve or lift one's mood. This link between sugar and mood is called the 'food–mood' link.

The best clinical study on carbohydrates and serotonin levels in the brain was published in 1972 in the well-known journal *Science*. The two researchers involved, Dr John Fernstrom and Dr Richard Wurtman, established scientifically for the first time that the protein and carbohydrate content of a meal can have a significant effect on the levels of different chemicals in the brain. Dr Wurtman has since proposed the theory that people who binge and overeaters seek out refined carbohydrate foods (foods containing white sugar and white flour) in an attempt to compensate for an underlying serotonin deficiency. When these people become depressed they may seek out refined carbohydrates in an attempt to boost their mood. This is the main theory proposing a definite link between bingeing on refined carbohydrates and elevation in mood, i.e. 'the food–mood link'.

Advice
Cut out all stimulants such as cola, caffeine, tea, coffee and sugar from the diet and take a high-potency B complex formula with at

least 50 mg of each of the B vitamins — Solgar makes a good formula called Megasorb Vitamin B complex -— to stabilise your energy.

Use only complex carbohydrates (brown rice, pasta, potatoes and wholewheat bread), and reduce refined carbohydrates (white sugar, white flour) to an absolute minimum.

Drink lots of bottled or filtered water instead of soft drinks. Avoid all processed foods as they are laden with additives — preservatives, colourants, flavourings and stabilisers. Some additives can affect the central nervous system directly, e.g. MSG (see above) is well known to cause migraine headaches.

You will therefore avoid mood-altering food and potentially harmful chemicals in the diet but will assist your eliminative organs, i.e. the skin, liver, kidney and bowel, considerably by sticking to a very natural diet of grains, fruit, vegetables, lean meats, water and herbal teas.

By using such a natural diet in the long term you will not just improve your energy and reduce food cravings but your feeling of well-being will be enhanced as well as your mood. In some patients, altering the diet alone is sufficient to treat anxiety or depression without the need for any medicines at all.

Case History — Angela: Age Thirty Years

Angela has very severe mood swings and low energy which used to occur for two to three days before her period but prior to coming to see me she noticed that her mood swings and fatigue were extending to ten days before her period and were more severe.

Angela's diet consisted of coffee with milk and sugar for breakfast, a muffin and a soft drink for lunch and a cooked meal often quite late in the evening; snacks consisted of crisps or chocolates. She used to have a very good diet but since a break-up with her boyfriend one year ago her eating habits deteriorated. She said that she felt depressed and didn't have the motivation to exercise or eat well any longer.

Angela was very aware of food and diet and so didn't need much education on nutrition; she was also aware that she was caught in a vicious cycle where the foods that she was consuming added to her low mood and produced cravings for the refined carbohydrates especially.

Merely by altering her diet by removing coffee, sugar, white flour and convenience foods, and altering her eating habits so that she had a substantial breakfast of muesli or oats with fresh fruit or yoghurt and ate the main meal in the middle of the day with just a light snack in the evening, and adding in a high-potency B complex supplement (which had 50 mg of each of the B vitamins), she showed a remarkable improvement.

If only people knew how important a role diet plays not just in their mood but in their physical well-being, they would not eat much of what our Western diet is made up of, i.e. processed, refined, chemical-laden foods. A more natural diet can improve central nervous system functions to the point where serotonin levels return to normal so returning one's mood to normal as well. Doing this alone may obviate the need for medicines completely.

Summary

Food is the best medicine of all. Many patients who fail to respond well to natural medicines often are eating incorrectly, i.e. they are either eating the wrong foods or eating at the wrong times of day and in a hurried way.

The more natural your diet the greater the likelihood that mood disturbances such as depression, irritability and anxiety have another origin and will respond well to natural medicines such as herbs or homoeopathics. It is now well accepted that one's mood can be altered quite significantly by foods that alter the levels of certain chemicals such as serotonin in the brain — this is referred to as the 'food–mood' connection. In an energy sense, certain foods such as coffee, caffeine and sugar will perk you up but will cause your energy level to drop afterwards so that you feel fatigued. In a similar way these foods also can lift your mood temporarily but can cause depression or anxiety afterwards.

Avoid refined carbohydrates (sugar and white flour and foods that contain these substances) as much as possible. Do not eat processed foods which have additives such as preservatives, colourants and flavourings, and reduce stimulants such as tea, coffee and caffeine in your diet. By doing this alone your mood will stabilise as you will be reducing the peaks and troughs in the levels of serotonin in the brain.

9

Nutritional Supplements

Overview of this Chapter

I have divided this chapter into four sections. The first section discusses the need for supplementation of the diet with vitamins and minerals; the second section deals with vitamins, principally the B vitamins; the third section covers minerals and in particular magnesium and calcium, as these are the two most important minerals for nervous function. The last section deserves special mention as it deals with amino acids (the building blocks of protein), some of which in high dosage have a very positive effect on anxiety, depression and insomnia. Some of these amino acids are so beneficial that they actually deserve a special chapter on their own.

Section 1: Introduction to Nutritional Supplements

Nutrients

There are six important nutrients that you need to keep your body healthy — carbohydrates, proteins, fats, vitamins, minerals and water.

The first three of these — carbohydrate, protein and fats — are called macronutrients since you need them in large quantities; hence they form the bulk of the diet.

Vitamins and minerals are termed micronutrients as you need only small amounts of them on a daily basis. Vitamins and minerals are essential for growth, vitality and well-being and save for a few exceptions cannot be manufactured by your body. Therefore, we must obtain them from food or via supplements.

Do You Need Vitamin/Mineral Supplements?
There is much debate about this issue among scientists, doctors and patients. It is best as in any controversial issue to study the arguments and then adopt a commonsense approach.

1. THE MEDICAL/SCIENTIFIC ARGUMENT
Most doctors and scientists would argue that supplementation with vitamins and minerals for most patients is unnecessary and merely a money-making exercise on the part of natural medicine companies. They would argue, as I did for some time, that a good diet with lots of fruit, vegetables and whole foods will provide sufficient micronutrition. Most doctors would also argue that the RDAs (recommended daily allowances), set down by a group of government scientists, are adequate to avoid the classic deficiency diseases (scurvy, pellagra, beriberi, etc.) and so anyone taking the RDA of each micronutrient should not have symptoms of vitamin/mineral deficiencies.

Having been trained as a scientist and a medical doctor, I understand where they are coming from and have agreed with their argument for many years. In the last ten years, however, I have read much and attended many seminars on nutritional medicines and have come to realise that the medical/scientific argument does not hold water any more.

2. THE ARGUMENT OF NUTRITIONISTS, NATUROPATHS, HOMOEOPATHS, ETC.
Many professionals working in the field of natural medicine would argue that vitamin/mineral supplementation is absolutely essential. They base this argument on the fact that:
- much of the modern diet consists of processed food

- a lot of the macronutrients (vegetables, fruits, carbohydrates, etc.) are grown in nutritionally depleted soils, and
- most doctors and scientists are not trained in nutritional medicine and so know very little about this topic.

Having studied both orthodox and natural medicine, I have little doubt that in today's world vitamin/mineral supplementation is necessary. Most processed and convenience foods are for the most part devoid of essential micronutrients; they are also energy-deficient. In addition, if you buy most of your fruit and vegetables at a supermarket in a modern city, you can be pretty sure that these foods are deficient as they are grown in market garden areas on the outskirts of the city in soil that is often very depleted. Because of the economic pressure put on market gardeners to supply the steady demand of city dwellers, the soil is not left for long enough to recuperate but rather must sustain one crop after another. Because many of these foods are sprayed with pesticides, these chemicals enter the soil and damage it (not to speak of the damage that they do when they enter your body when you eat these vegetables and fruits).

Most doctors and scientists know little about nutrition and even less about nutritional supplements. Very recently, my son David was in hospital. In the bed next to him was a nine-year-old girl whose mother was very knowledgeable about natural medicine; she was using homoeopathic medicine to assist the child to recover from an operation. The surgeon who had operated on her daughter came in as she and I were having a conversation about MSG (monosodium glutamate), a flavour enhancer added to many foods today. She asked the surgeon what he thought about MSG. His answer was: 'I never heard of MSG. What is it?' Hence, be careful when you ask your GP or medical specialist about vitamin/mineral supplements; the truth is you may be much more knowledgeable than they.

If you need convincing about the value of supplementation there are many scientific articles in the literature to validate its importance. In the 1950s Dr Abram Hoffer and Dr Humphrey

Osmond in the USA began treating schizophrenia with high doses of vitamin B3 (niacin). Their studies showed that niacin, in combination with standard medical therapy, doubled the number of recoveries in a one-year period.

Intravenous magnesium sulphate (magnesium is an essential mineral) is given in some hospitals to heart attack patients to speed recovery time.

Chromium (a trace mineral) is now known to help regulate the blood sugar level and so is useful in patients with diabetes and hypoglycaemia.

Vitamins and Minerals are Critical for Good Health

As I stated above, carbohydrate, protein and fats provide you with energy. To release this energy from these foods, micronutrients (vitamins and minerals) are needed.

If you imagine that your body is an internal combustion engine (car engine), that the macronutrients are the fuel or petrol and that vitamins and minerals are the spark plugs, then you will understand how these micronutrients actually work. Vitamins and minerals are vital for numerous enzyme or chemical reactions that control our metabolism. Zinc, for example, is essential in over 200 enzyme reactions in the body; hence a deficiency in zinc can have wide-ranging effects. You can now see how a deficiency in even one vitamin or mineral can endanger your health.

Essential Nutrients

By 'essential nutrients' I mean those micronutrients which your body *cannot* manufacture and which therefore must be obtained from the diet or from supplements. Table 9.1 lists some of these.

Table 9.1

Essential vitamins	Essential minerals	Essential amino acids
Fat-soluble —		
Vitamin A	Calcium	L-isoleucine
Vitamin D	Magnesium	L-leucine
Vitamin E	Phosphorus	L-valine

Vitamin K	Iron	L-methionine
	Zinc	L-threonine
Water-soluble —		
Vitamin C	Copper	L-phenylalanine
Vitamin B_1	Manganese	L-tryptophan
Vitamin B_2	Iodine	
Vitamin B_3	Chromium	**Essential fatty acids**
Vitamin B_5	Potassium	Linoleic acid
Vitamin B_6	Sodium	Linolenic acid
Vitamin B_{12}		Oleic acid
Folic acid		Arachidonic acid
Biotin		

How Vitamins and Minerals Work Together

Vitamins and minerals regulate the conversion of food to energy in the body. See Figure 9.1.

Figure 9.1

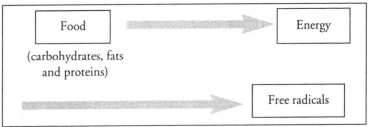

Most of the food you eat is broken down in the small intestine and then absorbed into the bloodstream. It is carried in the portal vein to the liver, where it is broken down by enzymes to release energy. In the process of converting food to energy, free radicals are produced that can damage the body and, if not got rid of, can set the stage for degenerative diseases such as heart disease, arthritis, premature ageing and cancer.

In the release of energy from the foods we eat, the B complex vitamins and magnesium are crucial. These micronutrients often work as a team, the presence of one enhancing the function of the other. See Figure 9.2.

Figure 9.2

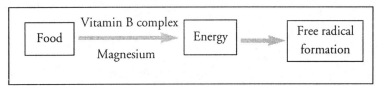

Other micronutrients act to protect the body from the potential damage of free radicals. Vitamins A, C and E and the minerals selenium, zinc and manganese play a vital role in damage limitation and so prevent the onset of degenerative diseases. These three vitamins and three minerals also work as a team, enhancing each other's protective effects. This is illustrated in Figure 9.3.

Figure 9.3

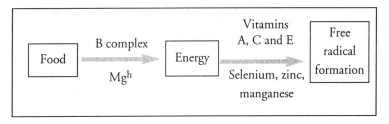

Section 2: Vitamins and Tranquilliser Use

In the first part of this chapter we spoke about the general role of supplements. Now I wish to deal with specific vitamins and minerals which relate to people who have used, or are using, tranquillisers.

All the B complex vitamins are water-soluble. Therefore, any excess is excreted from the body via the kidneys. Since an excess intake of any of the B complex vitamins will not be stored in the body, toxicity is very rare. Extremely high doses can cause transient side effects, but normal doses are very safe. Supplement with B complex when you are under stress, on the pill, pregnant, or eating a diet rich in sugary foods. Since B complex are often derived from yeast, brewers' yeast is a good source of all of these vitamins.

Vitamin B_1 (Thiamine)
Thiamine is known as the 'moral vitamin' because it has such a beneficial effect on the nervous system and on mental attitude. This vitamin like all the B complex vitamins is best used as a B complex formula and *not* alone. Any excess which is taken in food or as a supplement is not stored in the body and so toxicity is rare. It is destroyed by heat used in cooking.

Thiamine is important for growth and for digestion, especially digestion of carbohydrates. Its main role is keeping the nervous system and muscles functioning normally. A deficiency of thiamine causes beriberi. The best natural sources of this vitamin are dried yeast, rice husks, wholewheat, oatmeal, most vegetables and milk.

Vitamin B_2 (Riboflavin)
This is the most common vitamin deficiency in the Western world. Like thiamine, riboflavin is water-soluble and so any excess is excreted via the kidneys. Unlike thiamine, it is *not* destroyed by heat; rather it is damaged by light. For this reason milk is sold in cartons nowadays rather than glass bottles.

Riboflavin is important in the metabolism of carbohydrates, fats and proteins. Like B_1, it aids growth and reproduction and in addition it promotes healthy skin, nails and hair. Vitamin B_2 can help eliminate sores on the mouth, lips and tongue. The best natural sources are yeast, milk, liver and green leafy vegetables. A deficiency leads to lesions on the mouth, lips, skin and genitalia.

Vitamin B_6 (Pyridoxine)
This is actually a group of substances — pyridoxine, pyridoxinal and pyridoxamine — that work together. This vitamin must be present for the production of antibodies and red blood cells. Some of the 'good' bacteria in the bowel make B_6. This is the reason

why some patients show up as having a low red cell count on blood tests. One commonly used medical blood test is called a 'full blood count' and in the past I often picked up a low red cell count but couldn't account for it as all the other red cell indicators were normal. Prior to learning about the role of the vitamins, I disregarded this reading as unimportant. Today, being a bit more knowledgeable, I advise such patients to take a B complex supplement.

A deficiency of this vitamin can cause anaemia, glossitis (inflamed tongue) and seborrhoeic dermatitis.

NB Diabetics should be careful when using B_6 as this vitamin can decrease the need for insulin, causing hypoglycaemia (low blood sugar level) if the dosage of insulin is not adjusted.

Vitamin B_6 also interacts with levodopa, used to treat Parkinson's disease.

The oral contraceptive pill can result in a deficiency of this vitamin so if you are on the pill make sure that you supplement with pyridoxine. The RDA is 2–2.5 mg but many over-the-counter preparations have anything from 5 mg to 500 mg. Do not use doses over 500 mg as very high doses can cause neurological disorders. A good guide that the dosage of B_6 is too high is night restlessness and very vivid dreams.

Vitamin B_6 acts as a natural diuretic; it also reduces muscle spasm and leg cramps as well as preventing various nervous and skin disorders. Good natural sources of vitamin B_6 include brewers' yeast, wheat bran, wheatgerm and liver.

Vitamin B_3 (Niacin)
The first evidence relating a nutritional deficiency to mental disturbances emerged when it was found that pellagra — which results in depression and dementia — could be cured by niacin supplements. Many experiments have now shown that some symptoms of mental illness can be switched on and off by altering vitamin levels in the body.

Dr Shulman, reporting in the *British Journal of Psychiatry*, found that forty-eight out of fifty-nine psychiatric patients had a folic acid deficiency. Other research has shown that the majority of the mentally and emotionally ill are deficient in one or more of the B vitamins or vitamin C. Even normal, happy people can become anxious or depressed when made folic acid or niacin deficient.

Niacin is essential for the synthesis of sex hormones (oestrogen, progesterone and testosterone) as well as cortisone and thyroxine; it is also necessary for a healthy nervous system. Niacin can be manufactured in the body from the amino acid tryptophan; hence it is not an essential vitamin.

As noted above, a deficiency in niacin causes pellagra, which is described by the three 'Ds' — diarrhoea, depression and dementia. The RDA is 12–18 mg but you will find between 50 and 100 mg in a good formulation. Good natural sources include liver, meat, fish and wholegrains.

Case History

I remember one particular patient that I had in South Africa who had virtually untreatable halitosis (bad breath). We tried a fermentation control diet, supplementation with acidophilus and whey, restoration of leucine in the diet and a whole range of other treatments. Nothing seemed to work. In desperation I used 100 mg of niacin twice daily; to my surprise three weeks later her breath was back to normal. This case reminded me of the fact that niacin can help eliminate bad breath. Interestingly, it can also reduce the severity of migraine attacks.

Choline

This substance is also a member of the B complex family of vitamins. It is one of the few substances able to penetrate the blood brain barrier which protects the brain against variations in daily diet. It goes directly into the brain cells to produce a chemical that aids memory. Hence it is important in overcoming the problem of memory loss in the elderly. It has been found that patients with Alzheimer's disease are deficient in a neurotransmitter called acetylcholine. Ingestion of more choline can prevent existing acetylcholine from being broken down.

In addition, choline combines with inositol, another B complex member, to form lecithin. Both choline and inositol can emulsify cholesterol so that it doesn't settle on artery walls or in the gall bladder to form stones.

Natural sources of choline include egg yolks, yeast, liver, brain, heart, green leafy vegetables.

The RDA for choline has not yet been established. Use doses from 500 mg to 1,000 mg daily. The average B complex supplement has approximately 50 mg of choline.

Section 3: Minerals

Magnesium

This is known as the anti-stress mineral. As you learned earlier in this chapter, magnesium along with the B complex vitamins is important in the release of energy from food. Since a significant amount of this energy is needed by the nervous system, the brain in particular, magnesium is essential for nerve functions. See Figure 9.4.

Figure 9.4

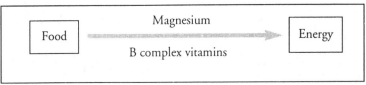

An overactive nervous system or overstressed body will become depleted of magnesium and B complex. Hence the recommendation to increase your intake of these micronutrients during times of stress.

People with addictions, to alcohol and tranquillisers especially, are often deficient in magnesium. This mineral is also helpful in fighting depression.

Dosage: RDA is 300–350 mg. Doses of 400 mg may cause diarrhoea. It is best taken with calcium; in fact dolomite is a good source of magnesium as it has half as much magnesium as calcium. Magnesium supplements should be taken alongside calcium but with twice as much calcium as magnesium; magnesium is essential for calcium metabolism. They work in harmony to maintain cardiovascular health. If you are taking magnesium on its own I would recommend a product called Slow Mag (Merck), a slow-release form of magnesium. Use one to two tablets morning and evening.

Calcium
Calcium is the best-known mineral in that most parents are aware that it is important for strong bones and healthy teeth in growing children and so prevents rickets and osteomalacia. Many women also know that when the level of oestrogen drops during menopause the bones can lose calcium and so become brittle (osteoporosis). Almost all of the body's calcium is found in the bones and teeth. In order for calcium to be absorbed from the food you eat, you must have sufficient vitamin D. Large quantities of fat, phytic acid (found in grains) and oxalic acid (found in chocolate and rhubarb) are capable of preventing calcium absorption in the bowel.

Teenagers with growing pains often get relief by increasing their intake of calcium, as do women who suffer from menstrual cramps.

Calcium is important not just for strong bones and teeth but for keeping your heartbeat regular. It also alleviates insomnia, helps the body metabolise iron and aids the nervous system, especially with nerve impulse transmission. The RDA is 800–1,200 mg. Remember that calcium and iron are the two minerals most deficient in a typical Western woman's diet.

Some authorities are concerned that increased calcium

supplementation may result in an increased risk of calcium oxalate kidney stones. Calcium citrate reduces this risk as some of the citrate's effects inhibit the formation of kidney stones. Hence calcium citrate is probably the best form of calcium salt to use.

Section 4: Amino Acids

Amino acids are relatively new nutritional supplements in that it is only in the last few decades that we have come to recognise how beneficial some of these can be in the treatment of various conditions. Some such as glycine, alanine and glutamic acid have been found to be very effective in the treatment of benign enlargement of the prostate gland in men; others such as phenylalanine have both painkilling and antidepressant effects while tryptophan is a supreme anti-anxiety medicine.

Amino acids are the building blocks from which protein is made. They form part of our food and the protein content is then broken down in the small intestine into individual amino acids. Some of these amino acids are very important for the synthesis of neurotransmitters in the brain. Neurotransmitters are chemicals that pass messages from one nerve cell to the next, i.e. they transmit information from nerve cell to nerve cell in the brain.

Figure 9.5

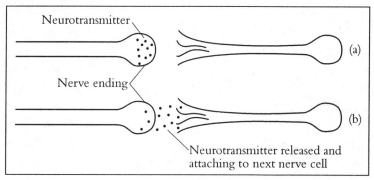

107

Examples of these neurotransmitters are dopamine, acetylcholine, serotonin and noradrenalin. Too much or too little of these neurotransmitters can have a significant effect on mood, anxiety level and sleep patterns. Many conventional drugs for the central nervous system such as Prozac or Zoloft alter the levels of these neurotransmitters in an attempt to enhance mood. Depression has been associated with low levels of serotonin and so drugs such as Prozac aim to increase serotonin levels and in so doing elevate mood as well.

Some amino acids, such as tryptophan, are used by the brain to manufacture serotonin and so the higher the blood levels of tryptophan the greater the amount of serotonin produced in the brain. Let's begin by looking in a bit more detail at how some of these amino acids work.

L-Tryptophan
This is the precursor of a very important neurotransmitter, serotonin, in the brain. For tryptophan to be converted to serotonin, certain B vitamins and magnesium are necessary. See Figure 9.6.

Figure 9.6

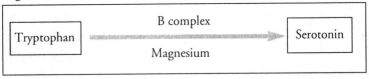

Tryptophan is a fascinating amino acid as it has been proven beneficial in the treatment of anxiety, depression, insomnia and alcoholism. Tryptophan-rich foods include cottage cheese, milk and all protein foods such as fish, nuts and meat. However, this amino acid has to be used in high dosage for it to have a therapeutic effect.

It normally comes in tablets of either 250 mg or 500 mg. The recommended dosage is 500 mg three times daily. If using this or any other amino acid always take it away from food and with a little fruit juice.

This amino acid, tryptophan, has been tested extensively at the Maryland Psychiatric Research Center in the USA and has been shown to be of therapeutic value in the treatment of depression and anxiety. Unlike the BZs and antidepressant drugs, there is no danger of addiction or overdose. Tryptophan is side-effect-free in that it is a purely natural constituent of our diet and so the body does not have to change any function to make use of it.

It is best taken with certain B vitamins, in particular niacin (B_3) and pyridoxine (B_6), and magnesium. (In fact, all amino acids should be taken with a B complex supplement.) The antidepressant effect of tryptophan can be profound if it is taken in a 2:1 ratio with niacin, e.g. 500 mg of tryptophan and 250 mg of niacin. In addition, niacin has an antidepressant effect of its own.

Phenylalanine

This is a natural 'upper' in that it elevates mood and mental well-being. It is taken up by the brain and converted into dopamine and noradrenalin, both of which increase mental alertness and vitality. Dopamine and noradrenalin are called excitatory neurotransmitters in that they excite the brain by stimulating the centres of alertness, memory and mood; they also increase sexual interest. As a result, phenylalanine has therapeutic benefit in the treatment of depression, low vitality, poor memory and decreased libido. It should *not* be used if you are pregnant, have high blood pressure, have phenylketonuria or skin cancer. Phenylalanine is readily available in 250–500 mg tablets. For the treatment of depression use 500 mg between meals, i.e. three times daily, and as with all amino acids take it with a little fruit juice.

It is best to take vitamin C — about 2,000 mg daily — along with phenylalanine, as the latter needs vitamin C to be converted into dopamine and noradrenalin. This is illustrated in Figure 9.7.

Figure 9.7

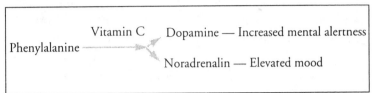

Tyrosine

Tyrosine is yet another amino acid that has proven valuable in the treatment of nervous disorders. Clinical studies have shown it to have a beneficial therapeutic effect in the treatment of depression and anxiety. Tyrosine has helped cocaine addicts conquer their habit by helping them cope with the withdrawal effects of fatigue, depression and irritability. In fact, it is helpful in withdrawal from not only cocaine but a number of recreational drugs including amphetamines.

Tyrosine should be taken with a high-potency B complex supplement and vitamin C. Take 500 mg twice daily between meals with a little fruit juice.

I have summarised the information in this section in Table 9.2.

Table 9.2

Amino acid	Converted in the brain into	Used to treat	Dosage
Tryptophan	Serotonin	1. Anxiety 2. Depression	500 mg 3 x daily
Phenylalanine	Dopamine and noradrenalin	1. Low vitality 2. Depression	500 mg 3 x daily
Tyrosine	Dopamine and noradrenalin	1. Withdrawal from drugs 2. Depression	500 mg 2 x daily

Summary

Despite what some scientists and doctors say, vitamin and mineral supplementation is very important in today's world. This is because the modern diet is rich in processed foods which often are devoid of essential micronutrients, and in addition, fruits and vegetables that we consume are often grown in depleted soils.

For nervous disorders, the two most important supplements are B complex vitamins and a calcium magnesium combination.

Three amino acids in high dosage have been shown to have therapeutic value in the treatment of depression and anxiety. Since tryptophan is used by brain cells to manufacture serotonin, tryptophan in high dosage can elevate one's mood and alleviate anxiety and insomnia. Phenylalanine is converted in the brain to dopamine and noradrenalin, which stimulate mental alertness, vitality, memory and mood. Phenylalanine is used therefore for depression and low vitality; it is best taken with vitamin C. Another amino acid, tyrosine, has been helpful in withdrawal from recreational drugs such as cocaine and amphetamines. All amino acids are best taken with a B complex supplement, between meals and with a little fruit juice.

Meditation, Relaxation and Other Self-Help Techniques

10

Introduction

This chapter is for people who do not want to take medicines — natural or unnatural — on an ongoing basis to treat their nervous and emotional difficulties. It is also for people who want to obtain a sense of peace and contentment in their lives, and for people who want to develop their true potential as human beings.

Because the neuro-endocrine system connects all parts of the body physically and therefore energetically as well, using more subtle techniques such as relaxation, meditation and visualisation can not only alleviate nervous disorders but lead you to a greater understanding of your true nature and allow the real *you* to emerge.

In this chapter I am going to discuss self-help techniques that you can use to alleviate stress and nervous tension. These techniques include meditation, deep relaxation, breathing, exercise, visualisation and biofeedback.

Silent Meditation

Because our world is full of activity, especially verbal activity, we seldom make time to balance this activity with periods of inactivity. This balance is essential for the proper functioning of the neuro-endocrine system and therefore of the whole body. Sleep is a period of relative physical inactivity but not non-physical inactivity, e.g. one's mind and emotions are often extremely active and some people can be very active physically also. Silent meditation is the way to balance the neuro-endocrine system.

Case History

While I was visiting a medical clinic in the USA some years ago, the doctor in charge was demonstrating the effect of silent meditation on the blood flow to the right and left hemispheres of the brain. The patient was a male business executive who was highly stressed. The electrodes attached to his head measured the blood flow to both sides of his brain. There was a very high flow to the left brain but little to the right brain. After thirty minutes of silent meditation there was an equal blood flow to both sides of the brain; this is the natural state.

The stress of modern life leads to an imbalance in activity in the two sides of the brain which in turn causes further stress on the more subtle aspects of our being. As a consequence, the caring, compassionate, intuitive, creative and loving side of our nature gets less expression. Because of our social conditioning, men tend to have more extreme imbalances than women. Silent meditation is essential for us all but it is the male species that would appear to be in much greater need.

Through silent meditation we are able to withdraw from our busy lives and through this withdrawal we can begin to gain insights into ourselves and how we are living our lives. The greater your understanding of your true self the more comfortable you will feel allowing this side of you expression and the more you can become this person. In this way, you will re-find yourself and gain a deep peace and contentment in doing so; you *come home.* When you come home there is no more role playing, no game playing, no need to pretend or lie. You can bare yourself to the world without fear. Getting to know, becoming intimate with and learning to love your real self is the only means to happiness and the only way permanently to overcome anxiety, tension, fear, guilt and lack of anything (love, money, power . . .) in your life. The more finely tuned you are to yourself the more finely tuned you'll be to everyone and everything around you. You will sense the inner conflict in people more acutely, you will sense the anxiety, anger and frustration in others with ease; conversely, you'll also see the beauty and love in people and as a consequence will feel the urge to help them see it also.

Silent meditation is the key which unlocks the door to your soul, the real you. It is the single most important form of healing for people irrespective of religion, background, race or colour. Increasing one's level of self-awareness is the way out of difficulties on this planet; if each of us practises the art of silent meditation on a daily basis, there will be hope for humanity. Practise for a minimum of thirty minutes daily and if possible involve the rest of your family. In that way, you are less likely to be disturbed by your kids or spouse or partner.

Silent meditation is the single most important form of healing for all of us. Practise it daily.

Deep Relaxation

It is when we are deeply relaxed that healing occurs. If you cut your finger most of the healing will happen when you are deeply relaxed; chronic anxiety, over-activity, loss of sleep, stress and anything else which impairs your ability to relax deeply will slow this healing process, not only at a physical level but at all levels. You don't have to use your conscious mind to focus on the cut finger to enable it to heal; it heals automatically as if by magic. So healing is a natural process. Blocking this healing energy within oneself, through stress for example, is an unnatural process. Allow the magic of self-healing to occur by creating a space and time for you to relax deeply. First thing in the morning or last thing at night are perhaps the best times to do this; personally I prefer sunrise and sunset as these are the high-energy points of the day.

SELF-HEALING IS A NATURAL STATE.

There are many ways to relax deeply, from focusing on your breathing through progressive relaxation techniques, all the way through to self-hypnosis. The key with all of these techniques is to calm the body physically and mentally so that you can open up at a deeper level.

Breathing

Focusing your attention on something, to the exclusion of everything else, can have a calming effect. Focusing your attention on breathing is a powerful self-healing tool and an extraordinarily simple one — it is something that you can do anywhere, at any time and is remarkably effective.

Breathing is something you do not think about consciously; it is under the control of the involuntary nervous system. (I refer to this part of the nervous system as the adrenalin/noradrenalin system since adrenalin speeds you up and noradrenalin calms you down. One's day is supposed to be balanced by periods of activity — adrenalin release — and periods of rest and relaxation — noradrenalin release. Too much adrenalin or noradrenalin leads to an imbalance in the involuntary nervous system, causing problems with the sweat glands, heart rate, rate of breathing and depth of breathing.) During periods of stress, our rate and depth of breathing changes. Because of a high output of adrenalin, your breathing tends to be much faster and shallower. Because of the shallow breathing, you have to take a deep breath occasionally to maintain a normal level of oxygen in the bloodstream and cells of the body. People who are chronically stressed can often cope much better if they are taught to control their breathing. Here is a simple exercise that works well.

BREATHING EXERCISE
The purpose of this exercise is to breathe from your abdomen and to build up the level of carbon dioxide in the bloodstream, which has a strong relaxant effect.

Step 1. Push your tummy out as you begin inhaling, and when the tummy is expanded fully use your chest muscles to complete the in-breath.

Step 2. Practise this and when you are doing it with ease, inhale slowly through your nose. Hold your breath for five seconds and then breathe out quickly, expelling as much air as possible. Do this three times.

Step 3. Then take ten normal breaths, remembering to breathe from your abdomen.

Step 4. Repeat Step 2 but holding the breath for seven seconds instead of five.

Step 5. Then breathe normally again.

The more you practise this exercise, the more effective it will be at calming you down. This is a simple means of using your own power to control nervous symptoms — practise it daily and it will work for you.

THE MAGICAL SIDE OF BREATHING
Breathing is controlled by the involuntary nervous system but at will you can take conscious control and so alter the rate and depth of breathing. This is the only body function where this is possible. Most cultures on this planet regard breathing and eating as the two most important elements of good health. To function effectively the cells of your body need energy. They get this energy by breaking down food in the presence of oxygen.

Figure 10.1

Food + O_2 ----------▶ Release of energy

Each cell of your body, if it is to remain healthy, needs these two basic elements (food and oxygen) supplied on a continuous basis. No small wonder then that breathing plays such a major role in the health systems of many cultures on this planet.

Breathing is a link between mind and body. Practising the breathing exercise mentioned above has a calming effect on the mind as well as the body. Breathing links the body and the spirit too; in fact the word for breath in a number of languages (e.g. Latin: 'spiritus') means spirit. It is also a link between the voluntary and involuntary parts of the nervous system, the conscious and unconscious parts of our being. Breathing is therefore extraordinarily special. Yogis in India are able to control their heart rate, blood pressure and bowel peristalsis simply by regulating their breath. Buddhist monks often learn the art of meditation by first focusing on their breathing, since this can change one's level of consciousness — slow, deep breathing has a calming effect while fast, shallow breathing makes one more anxious.

For the above reasons, it is important to practise deep breathing daily and to begin a relaxation and meditation session with deep inhalations and fully exhaling.

Exercise

Exercise is the natural state. I grew up in the countryside where life was very simple and I was very physically active. The local village was two miles away and as a child I often walked to primary school and home again in the afternoon. I would walk or cycle regularly to buy groceries for my mother and didn't think much about it. Since going to university in my late teens and early twenties, I became much more sedentary, often sitting in libraries for days on end studying.

In the modern world, people do not have to exert themselves physically, i.e. they don't have to walk or run long distances as there are cars and motorcycles, they don't have to fetch water as there is a mains supply and so on. Today we spend most of our time sitting — while at work, in a car, on a train, etc. As a consequence, we now find that we have to create a period in our day when we can exercise, to maintain a semblance of the natural state.

When I was a child I was not consciously aware that I was exercising when I was cycling around the roads, or climbing mountains, or walking to the village. It was fun. Today people take exercising too seriously and turn it into a drudgery. The key to gaining physical fitness is to have 'fun'. The fittest squash players I've met have been young guys who go to discos and night clubs to dance; they become fit enough to compete in sport at a very high level and have lots of fun dancing. What form of physical activity do you enjoy that is fun for you?

Exercise should not be about jogging, or running, or whatever, for a set period every day. There is no imagination, creativity or fun in that. Your mind will focus on the time element and you'll want to get the session over and done with as soon as possible. Rather focus on having fun dancing, trampolining, mountain climbing, cycling with friends or family, and have little games or competitions to make it more interesting. Watch how children play; they are intensely focused on what they're doing, oblivious to time.

PHYSICAL EXERCISE MUST BE FUN!

BENEFITS OF EXERCISE

Regular exercise leads to an increased ability to cope with stress by:

- improving heart function — exercise reduces heart rate and blood pressure as well as improving heart muscle tone
- reducing the output of adrenalin and cortisone from the adrenal glands in response to stress
- improving the oxygen uptake of all cells in the body

- improving self-esteem and feeling of well-being
- increasing energy levels

The last statement is particularly pertinent as many people refuse to exercise because they don't have enough energy; however, they will never have the energy unless they exercise. Remember that exercising is a bit like breathing; it is a natural state so just do it without thinking too much about it. Go dancing, walking, jogging, running, or whatever you feel like doing today, and *enjoy* it!

EXERCISE INCREASES YOUR ENERGY LEVELS AND GIVES YOU A SENSE OF WELL-BEING. IT IS AN EXCELLENT DE-STRESSER.

Visualisation

This is one of the most powerful and most underutilised abilities we have. Creating visual images has a potent effect on our physiology and our emotional state. For example, if you have a fear of spiders and you visualise a spider beside you where you are right now, your heart will beat faster, your breathing will become faster and you'll begin to sweat (changes in physiology); in addition, you may experience great anxiety to the point of screaming (changes in emotional state).

Most people think and learn in images. Stories, plays, poems and songs all create images which may be different for each of us. The song 'The Young Ones' by Cliff Richard reminds me of a summer's day when I was preparing to go fishing; the poem 'The Stolen Child' by W.B. Yeats reminds me of a pub in Ballyvaughan, Co. Clare. Imagery is an integral part of our being. We can create images of how we would like to be in the future and because these images have a direct effect on our physical and emotional bodies, they alter us in a way that allows the image to become real.

The work of Dr Carl Simonton and his wife, Stephanie Matthews-Simonton, with cancer patients has been an inspiration to everyone in the business of healing. From experience with hundreds of patients at their world-famous Cancer Counseling and Research Center in Dallas, Texas, the Simontons have demonstrated time and again the power of relaxation and visualisation to overcome cancer; they have described in their book *Getting Well Again* (London, Bantam: 1978) how positive visual images and increased self-awareness can contribute to survival in cancer patients.[1] Since their pioneering work in the 1970s, visualisation and guided imagery have become much more popular and accepted healing tools. There are many fine books to read on this topic but my favourite is *Creative Visualisation* by Shakti Gawain (San Rafael (CA), New World Library: 1979). If you haven't read this book or practised the wonderful exercises in visualisation that she mentions, I would urge you to do so as soon as possible.

Visualisation can be used for any illness and can also be used to achieve whatever you want to achieve in your life. By creating a visual image or goal you are making it happen by believing that it is possible. You then automatically remove any blocks preventing it from happening.

Problems with Visualisation

When I first started to use this technique with patients, I was amazed to find that some people were unable to visualise. Clearly, some people are more visual than others. Some people feel or sense things rather than see them; others think in words. We are all different. Through this process of imagery, I have found that

---

[1]   Dr Simonton first used the visualisation technique in 1971 with a patient who had incurable cancer. Three times a day the patient practised a visualisation technique which involved visualising his cancer as a group of weak, confused cells, growing out of control, and his white blood cells as highly organised soldiers attacking and destroying the cancer cells. He visualised his body removing the dead cells, his energy increasing and a feeling of well-being returning. The incurable patient overcame his cancer and is still alive today.

changes begin to occur, i.e. a person who was very visual may begin to feel or sense more and vice versa. Hence it is not necessary to be visual to practise visualisation. Seeing a spider in one's mind's eye has much the same result as feeling its presence.

Most people have some degree of difficulty with focusing on the 'desired outcome' when their immediate circumstances seem overwhelming. For example, it is difficult to imagine yourself a millionaire when you are struggling to survive, or it is difficult to imagine your tumour shrinking when you are aware of the pain or discomfort it is causing you. However, you have to create space and time on a frequent basis to channel positive energy towards your body's healing process. Not to channel energy towards or not to believe in the desired outcome is guaranteeing that the opposite will happen. It is as simple as that. If I play a game of tennis with someone and I do not believe that I can win the match, then I will not fight and struggle to win and so the outcome is inevitable; the harder the struggle, the greater the sense of achievement in winning.

Biofeedback

Biofeedback is learning how to regulate a person's body functions to reduce physical and psychological stress. It involves the use of a biofeedback machine which records a person's physiological responses to stress, e.g. heart rate, blood pressure, body temperature and so on. The person is then taught a simple relaxation technique such as those described earlier in this chapter and he/she can then see the effect this has on those same physiological responses. This encourages the person to use the relaxation technique as he/she has visual proof of its effectiveness. Biofeedback can be used to reduce muscle tension — particularly in the neck and lower back, lower one's heart rate and blood pressure, increase body temperature — especially where the hands and feet are cold, and improve digestive functions, as stress often has a negative effect on the gastro-intestinal tract.

In Ireland I had a patient who had all the classic signs of anxiety — increased heart rate (ninety-six per minute), high blood pressure, icy cold hands and feet, digestive problems and insomnia. He had been treated by his GP with tranquillisers and psychotherapy over a period of six months with little success. He came to me out of desperation as I was usually the last port of call for patients at that time; as my reputation grew I slowly became the first or second port of call, which pleased me enormously! I treated John with kava kava to help him cope better with his symptoms and referred him for biofeedback as he was quite young and had a fascination with machinery, and the tests that I did on him suggested that biofeedback and good breathing techniques and meditation would benefit him. I referred him to a therapist in Dún Laoghaire for the biofeedback and to my own meditation teacher for the rest. When I reviewed him six weeks later, his symptoms were greatly improved; after a further six weeks he was off all medication and symptom-free.

Biofeedback, when it is combined with relaxation, visualisation or meditation, can be very effective. In the USA at the Menninger Clinic in Topeka, Kansas, biofeedback training and brainwave therapy are used as a revolutionary treatment for drug or alcohol addiction. Biofeedback is used to demonstrate the effects of relaxation on the body. This relaxation response is then taken a step further with patients being helped to enter a very deep state of relaxation and once in this state to use visualisation techniques to enable them to see themselves rejecting drugs or alcohol. The third part of the treatment involves helping the patient reprogramme old behaviour patterns that led to drug abuse in the first instance. The programme also includes instruction in relapse prevention, shame and guilt work, self-development and self-help groups. Professor Paul Kulkosky, co-developer of the programme, reports a 70 per cent success rate after five years compared with only a 20 per cent success rate using traditional methods of medication plus psychotherapy. 'It's the most amazing thing to witness,' he says. 'The patients look younger after the programme of treatment and may have gone back to work or college or some have gotten jobs for the first time. They're just different people.'

It is wonderful to see positive changes like this occur in people's lives. It shows that where there is love and compassion on the part of the therapist and determination on the part of the patient, nothing is impossible. Biofeedback has now become part of many treatment programmes. Several studies have found that children suffering from hyperactivity and attention deficit disorder show improvement in academic performance when trained in biofeedback and relaxation techniques.

Summary

Silent meditation, deep relaxation and breathing techniques are all-powerful at alleviating anxiety and stress. They are techniques which are becoming more and more important for the Western urban person who leads an increasingly hectic life. It is important for such people to balance periods of high physical and mental activity with periods of complete inactivity as in silent meditation.

Another excellent de-stresser at the end of a busy day is exercise in some shape or form. It is important that the form of exercise chosen should be fun for you. Exercise allows one to release tensions built up during the day so that the tension does not become 'trapped' in the physical body.

Biofeedback is yet another means of controlling the effects of stress on the body by demonstrating to patients that they have control over the generation of symptoms. In some of the drug treatment centres around the world, biofeedback is combined with visualisation, deep relaxation and meditation to great effect.

11 *Practical Advice*

Having read the book, you are now either very knowledgeable or very confused. The purpose of this chapter is to convert much of the academic knowledge gained in the previous chapters into a usable form. I have covered only the more common conditions such as anxiety, depression and insomnia and used a step-by-step approach to help you cope with these conditions in a self-help manner but this does not substitute for seeing a professional health care practitioner.

Please keep in mind that for many reasons it is important to get off conventional drugs, primarily for your own sake but also for the sake of your children. Our children are getting the message from our generation that it is okay to use drugs, legal or illegal, when in emotional difficulty or when suffering from a nervous disorder. This has to change and the change has to start now with you and me. For the sake of the whole society seek a more natural way to assist yourself and most of all do not run away from deep-seated pain; rather confront the pain and grow as a human being from it, as this after all is the purpose of pain, i.e. it is there to help us to heal at a very deep level.

A lady came to see me in Capetown one day from Bloemfontein in the Orange Free State who was suffering from allergic sinusitis — I run special clinics for patients with severe allergic conditions mainly because of the work that I have done on asthma. At one point during the consultation she reached over to get her handbag and as she did so I could see numbers tattooed on her forearm. I knew that there were only two concentration camps that did this during the Second World War and she had been to Auschwitz. She had spent three years in this camp as a child having seen all her family being murdered by the Nazis. She did not know on a daily basis if she was going to live or die. She knew what fear was all about but refused to let it destroy her. This lady is one of the most inspirational people I have ever spoken to. She has healed the very deep wounds of her past, has forgiven the people who made her life a living hell and has now moved on. The fact that this lady is alive and well today is a statement of her own inner strength but to be able to forgive those who have caused her so much pain is a reflection of her own development as a human being. President Nelson Mandela was also able to forgive those who imprisoned him for twenty-seven years of his life and is now a wonderful human example of how important it is to heal oneself and to move on in life rather than living with the wounds of the past. I was brought up in a deeply divided society in Northern Ireland where hate and anger still control people's lives simply because we would rather live in the past than forgive and try to live in harmony with one another; the beautiful thing about being in South Africa despite all its difficulties is that this country was also very deeply divided but is now trying to heal its past and allow hope to enter the picture after over forty years of apartheid. There are now signs that there is real hope for a lasting peace in Northern Ireland too. Change is happening here and is precipitating similar changes elsewhere in the world.

I didn't realise how philosophical I was until I started to write this book. In truth, though, I am just very excited about the changes that are happening in different ways, especially in the area of medicine and healing, and I am happy to be a small part of that change and to nudge it along a wee bit. Below are some general guidelines to help you deal with the changes in your life; I hope you will see these changes in a positive light and help yourself through them as Nature intended.

Anxiety

The following step-by-step guide on how to deal with anxiety — whether acute or chronic — should be of help to you, either partially or completely, but if you are uncertain about what to do next consult your practitioner.

STEP 1: DIET

Alter your diet as follows:

(a) Cut out all refined carbohydrates — sugar as well as white flour.
(b) Cut out all stimulants — coffee, caffeine, tea, cola, etc.
(c) Add in more wholefoods such as brown bread, brown rice, brown pasta.
(d) Add in more vegetables and fruit.

STEP 2: NUTRITIONAL SUPPLEMENTS

Use supplements as follows:

(a) Vitamin B complex, 50 mg morning and evening for four weeks and then 50 mg once daily.
(b) Vitamin C, 2,000–4,000 mg daily in divided doses.
(c) Calcium and magnesium in a 2:1 ratio, i.e. twice as much calcium as magnesium — dolomite is a natural form of calcium and magnesium and no vitamin D is needed for assimilation. Five dolomite tablets are equivalent to 750 mg of calcium. Doses most often used are from 750 to 1,500 mg daily.
(d) Tryptophan, 500 mg twice daily between meals — not with milk or any other form of protein.

STEP 3: EXERCISE

Exercise to release any emotional or mental tensions. Do this for a minimum of twenty minutes daily as a routine. In addition use the breathing control technique described on p. 116 of this book.

If your anxiety level has not been reduced sufficiently doing the above then you must add in either a herbal or a homoeopathic medicine.

Herbal medicines. Use kava kava capsules (350 mg pure herb), one to two capsules three times daily.

Homoeopathic medicines. Use Ignatia, gelsemium or lycopodium in a 30c potency as drops or tablets. Use ten drops or one tablet six times daily for one day, and ten drops or one tablet three times daily afterwards, until an improvement in your condition is noticed. Homoeopathic medicines should be taken thirty minutes before or after anything strong-tasting in the mouth such as food, mint, peppermint or toothpaste, and should not be stored close to electrical devices such as computers, microwaves, etc.

You can use the homoeopathic or the herbal medicines separately or simultaneously, as you desire. Personally, I prefer to use one or the other depending on the sensitivity of the person, i.e. if the patient is a rather blocked, insensitive person I opt for the herbal as homoeopathics are less likely to work in such an individual, and if the person is quite open and sensitive I would be more likely to choose a homoeopathic, knowing that it is much more likely to work provided I choose the correct one.

STEP 5: DEAL WITH THE CAUSE FOR THE ANXIETY

It is important not to forget this despite how well you might be feeling on the above programme of treatment. The objective is to help you cope in the short term while you are dealing with the underlying cause, not to keep you on treatment for months or years. So, if it is within your power, solve the problem precipitating the anxious feelings. In this way you will get off all forms of medication and regain your health and happiness.

Insomnia

These steps are helpful for dealing with insomnia.

STEP 1: DIET

The biggest culprit in the diet is caffeine. Hence, cut out all foods containing caffeine such as coffee, cola drinks, tea, chocolate and chocolate drinks, cakes and biscuits as well as chocolate ice cream. Eat a diet rich in wholefoods and lots of fruit and vegetables and drink lots of water but not before bedtime.

STEP 2: EATING HABITS

Adopt good eating habits. By this I mean that it is better to eat the main meal in the middle of the day and to eat something quite light for supper. This is the way that I was brought up as a child but today things have changed such that many families are under so much pressure that they can often only get time to cook a main meal in the evening. There is a saying in English: 'Eat breakfast like a prince, eat lunch like a king and eat supper like a pauper', which basically advises us to put food into the body when it is most efficient, i.e. during the morning and afternoon, but to respect the fact that the body is preparing for sleep in the evening and not to burden it with a heavy digestive workload as this encourages the food to ferment in the bowel.

Another saying recommends: 'After dinner rest a while, after supper walk a mile', which is excellent advice, as you will learn just now.

STEP 3: DRUGS

A number of conventional medicines can cause insomnia as a side effect. These include many of the cough remedies, cold remedies which are available over the counter, oral contraceptives, beta blockers such as propranolol and atenolol, and asthmatic medicines such as Ventolin. Reduce the dosage or get off these drugs where possible but do so in consultation with a professional.

STEP 4: STRETCHING EXERCISES

Many people do not prepare for sleep. If you are anxious or you have been busy mentally, studying or working for example, create a transition period of twenty to thirty minutes in which you can unwind. This can take the form of stretching exercises to release muscle tension so that you are relaxed when going to bed. Another way of doing this is to get your partner to massage you. Going to bed when your mind is very busy is not conducive to a restful night's sleep.

STEP 5: BATHING/SHOWERING
A warm bath or shower will also help to ease muscle tension. I did not understand how important bathing was until a wise man who was also a healer advised me to use coarse sea salt in my bath and then to brush the skin working upwards from the feet stroking towards the heart. It is a way of cleansing the aura or energy field around the body. Personally, I have found it effective but do not get the time to do it every day.

STEP 6: PREPARING FOR SLEEP
While lying in bed it may be helpful to play some relaxing music or even a self-enhancement tape.

STEP 7: NUTRITIONAL SUPPLEMENTS
Refer to the section above on anxiety, as the same supplements are needed. However, as a sleep inducer L-tryptophan works best in a 500 mg dose along with vitamin B$_6$, 100 mg, niacin, 100 mg and chelated magnesium, 130 mg rather than a calcium magnesium supplement.

STEP 8: MEDICINE
The seven steps above are simple self-help measures well within your capability. If you have followed this advice and your insomnia persists then you need either a homoeopathic or a herbal medicine.

Herbal medicines:
1. If using kava kava, increase the evening dose from two to three capsules. If not using kava kava, start doing so.
2. If kava kava is not sufficiently effective by itself add

Dormeasan, which is manufactured by Bioforce; use twenty to thirty drops one hour before retiring and repeat at bedtime if necessary.

Homoeopathic medicines:

1. Valerianaheel is a remedy manufactured by Heel which also works well at the same dosage as Dormeasan.
2. There are a number of single homoeopathic remedies available for the treatment of insomnia but it is important to consult with a homoeopath to find the one most suitable for you.

Again I would advise using either a herbal or a homoeopathic separately; however, one can use the two in combination.

Depression

The steps below are helpful for mild to moderate depression but not for severe depression.

STEP 1: DIET

What I have written in the section above on anxiety is highly relevant here too as many refined carbohydrates have been linked with depression. Avoid hypoglycaemia (low blood sugar level) by eating small meals frequently.

STEP 2: NUTRITIONAL SUPPLEMENTS

(a) Vitamin B complex, 50 mg twice daily.

(b) Calcium and magnesium in a 2:1 ratio as in the supplement dolomite.

(c) It is important not to use calcium on its own as it can cause depression.

(d) Phenylalanine at a dosage of 500 mg three times daily between meals with a little fresh fruit juice.

(e) Zinc — 50 mg of elemental zinc daily taken in the evening with food.

STEP 3: EXERCISE

Try to do some form of enjoyable exercise for at least thirty minutes daily. Natural endorphins released in response to exercise produce a natural 'high'.

STEP 4: DRUGS

Steroids and oral contraceptives may cause the serotonin levels in the brain to drop, so causing depression. Long-term use of tranquillisers can also lead to depression. Wean yourself off these drugs if on them or avoid them where possible if you are not on them. Check with your doctor to ensure that thyroid function is normal (a decrease in function can cause depression).

STEP 5: MEDICINE

If the above simple self-help measures have not resulted in an improvement in your mood then you should use St John's Wort (Hypericum perforatum) in herbal or homoeopathic form.

Herbal medicines: Hypericum perforatum is the single most important natural antidepressant as it has proven its worth. Use it in herbal form at ten drops three times daily or one capsule (350 mg) two to three times daily. Personally, I prefer to use it three times daily and then after two to three weeks when its benefits become noticeable reduce to twice daily. Note, however, that it can take two to three weeks to produce an improvement in the condition.

Kava kava can also be used if there is accompanying anxiety. Use two capsules three times daily.

Homoeopathic medicines. Use hypericum in a 30c potency as tablets and suck one tablet six times daily for one day and then three times daily. As the mood improves reduce the dosage slowly, e.g. use it twice a day for a few days and then once a day for a few days and then stop it.

There are a number of other single homoeopathic remedies used in the treatment of depression but it is best to consult with a homoeopath to find the right remedy for you individually.

Coming Off Tranquillisers

STEP 1: DO IT GRADUALLY
Wean yourself off the drugs slowly — never stop suddenly!

STEP 2: GET HELP
Seek the help of a professional, preferably someone with experience in both conventional and alternative medicine.

STEP 3: FOLLOW GUIDELINES TO REDUCE DOSAGE
Reduce the dosage of the tranquilliser along the lines shown in Table 3.1 (see p. 32).

STEP 4: DIET
Eat a diet devoid of irritants to the central nervous system such as refined carbohydrates and stimulants. Eat a diet rich in wholefoods with lots of salads, fruits and vegetables. Stay on this diet for a minimum of six months.

STEP 5: NUTRITIONAL SUPPLEMENTS
(a) Vitamin B complex, 50 mg twice daily for six months and then once daily for six months.
(b) Vitamin C, 2,000–4,000 mg daily for six months and then half this dosage for six months.
(c) Tyrosine, 500 mg twice daily between meals with a little fresh fruit juice for six months.
(d) Calcium and magnesium — as described above under 'Anxiety' — for six months.

STEP 6: ACUPUNCTURE
This is the single most effective means of helping someone wean themselves off any drug that they may be addicted to. Find an acupuncturist with a good reputation who is capable of doing ear acupuncture (auriculo-therapy) and who has experience in helping with withdrawal.

STEP 7: MEDICINE

Herbal medicines. Use kava kava as dried herb — two capsules (350 mg pure herb) three times daily. Use hypericum as dried herb — one capsule (350 mg pure herb) three times daily. Use valerian and skullcap in tincture form — ten drops three times daily for the first three months; then use Nervol for a further three months.

Epilogue

I hope you enjoyed this book and that you have learned some things that will help make your life more enjoyable. Try where possible to stay drug-free and to teach your children by example, i.e. by showing them that the natural way is the only true way to heal.

I have tried to keep the text 'user-friendly' by minimising the number of technical terms and by lightening the factual detail with relevant case histories from my own practice.

If you have any comments that would enrich the book in any way feel free to write to me at the following address:

> PO Box 10632
> Glen Eagles
> 7945 Cape Town
> South Africa

I wish you peace and harmony and that you can radiate this peace to others. I also wish that you may glimpse the magic of Nature at work within your life.

The Restless Heart

Be still my restless heart
What is it that you fear;
I fear to die before I live,
There's so much in me I have to give
The shadows of doubt are near.

Thrum-thrum, thrum-thrum!
Like a loud and noisy drum;
There is no rest — there is no peace:
These restless yearnings do not cease;
Thrum-thrum! but come,
There is a sound above the drum — a different beat,
That plays another tune so sweet.

It calls to me — it speaks to me
With a haunting, tranquil melody;
It promises rest — it promises peace;
It promises that these yearnings will cease.
And above the drumbeat's din
I hear a voice — please let me in.

There's a gentle rap and a softer tap
On the door that leads to my heart;
Thrum-thrum! there starts the noisy drum,
But the different beat that is so sweet
Rises above the clamorous beat
Of the noisy drum.

The door to my heart is choked with weeds,
With no handle except from within;
And the gentle voice repeats — please let me in.
Only you can invite me into your heart,
Only you can open the door,
But outside I will wait with the patience of Love
Until your fears are no more.

There's a river of light before my eyes
And the handle within is clear,
Just turn it once and open the door
And see who is standing there.
Thrum-thrum! now starts the noisy drum
But the different beat that is so sweet
Drowns out the noisy beat
And all that remains is the tune so sweet.

Be still my heart — for Love is near,
There is no noise — there is no fear,
Just open the door and let Him in.
Now there is a different beat,
Another tune — a tune so sweet
It brings out the spring of life in me
For I know I cannot rest until I rest in Thee.

Index